D0929530

Heterosexism in Health and Social Care

Heterosexism in Health and Social Care

Julie Fish
De Montfort University

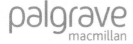

First published 2006 by
PALGRAVE MACMILLAN
Houndmills, Basingstoke, Hampshire RG21 6XS and
175 Fifth Avenue, New York, N.Y. 10010
Companies and representatives throughout the world

PALGRAVE MACMILLAN is the global academic imprint of the Palgrave Macmillan division of St. Martin's Press, LLC and of Palgrave Macmillan Ltd. Macmillan® is a registered trademark in the United States, United Kingdom and other countries. Palgrave is a registered trademark in the European Union and other countries.

ISBN-13: 978-1-4039-4123-7   hardback
ISBN-10: 1-4039-4123-8   hardback

This book is printed on paper suitable for recycling and made from fully managed and sustained forest sources.

A catalogue record for this book is available from the British Library.

Library of Congress Cataloging-in-Publication Data

Fish, Julie, 1955–
    Heterosexism in health and social care / Julie Fish.
        p. cm.
    Includes bibliographical references and index.
    ISBN 1-4039-4123-8 (hardback)
    1. Gays–Medical care. 2. Social work with gays. 3. Heterosexism. I. Title.

RA564.9.H65F57 2006
362.1086'64–dc22

2006046017

10   9   8   7   6   5   4   3   2   1
15 14 13 12 11 10 09 08 07 06

Printed and bound in Great Britain by
Antony Rowe Ltd, Chippenham and Eastbourne

For Annette
with love

Contents

List of Tables and Figures

Acknowledgements

Many of the ideas for this book are the result of my involvement with a number of community-based research projects which have informed my thinking about future directions for health and social care for lesbians, gay men and bisexual people. Health and social care activists and policy-makers have identified the importance of the development of an agenda for lesbian, gay and bisexual people's health and social care needs: many previous attempts have stalled due to the scale of the task. This book is intended as a contribution to this agenda – for policy-makers, lesbian, gay and bisexual activists, health and social care practitioners and students in these professions.

The study has derived support from many people, in particular, the lesbians who took part in focus group discussions or who completed the survey which form the second part of the book. They gave their time, shared their insights and their contributions act as exemplars of hetero-sexism in everyday interactions with service providers and provide illustrations of the ways that risk perceptions are framed by heterosexist concepts. These women must remain anonymous (and their identities are protected in the text by pseudonyms), but there are others (both people and organisations) without whom my 'impossible' target of 1000 lesbian survey participants would never have been reached.

I am very grateful to Sue Wilkinson who was generous with her feedback in supervising the PhD from which this book is partly drawn. The members of the BSA Lesbian Study Group have been an ongoing source of constructive criticism, especially Nicki Thorogood. I have benefited from the insights and work of Celia Kitzinger and Tamsin Wilton. Thanks go to Dave Ward, Head of School of Applied Social Sciences at De Montfort University for ongoing support. Discussions with Dipti Morjaria, Anjum Mouj, Annika Parisotto, Jane Anger and Katy Wright have provided useful counterpoints to my arguments. My thanks go to my parents for their own successes in coming out, on my behalf, to their friends and acquaintances.

Finally, I am indebted to my partner, Annette Greenwood, whose love, support and sense of humour sustained me through the writing of this book.

Permission to use excerpts from Rory Carroll's article was obtained from *The Guardian*.

Part I
Understanding Heterosexism in Health and Social Care

Part I

1
What is Heterosexism?

Understanding homophobia

It was a balmy evening and Old Compton Street was even more
crowded than usual. The drinkers spilling out from pubs onto the
pavement to catch the sun's dying rays were relaxed . . . Work was
over and for once the forecast was good for the bank holiday week-
end. At 6.37 p.m. it happened. A sound like a massive crunch. It split
the air, drowning out everything else. In less than a second, the
inside of the *Admiral Duncan* was transformed into a scene from
hell. A white flash, then a blast shook the building and hurtled hun-
dreds of nails everywhere. Windows splintered, showering shards.
Eyewitnesses said there were a couple of seconds of stunned silence
before the screams began. Through a cloud of dust and smoke stag-
gered dozens of bleeding, choking, mutilated people . . . It was as if a
madman had thrown a bucket of blood everywhere . . . (Carroll,
1999)

The bombing of the *Admiral Duncan* pub was the third in a series of
bombings in the spring of 1999 against 'minority' populations in London
by a member of a right-wing extremist organisation. The previous two
bombs, which targeted the Bangladeshi community in Brick Lane and
the African-Caribbean community in Brixton, had mercifully exploded
without loss of life. The third bomb had been planted to achieve maximum
carnage in Soho, London's lesbian and gay district: three people died
and many more were seriously injured. Such extreme forms of anti-gay
violence have come to be known as homophobic attacks on lesbian, gay,
bisexual and transgender communities and, in the case of the Soho bomb,
their heterosexual friends. Homophobia gives name to hate crimes (such

3

as so-called queer bashing), the bullying of young lesbians and gay men in schools, the killing of David Morley – himself a survivor of the Soho bomb – and recently, of Jody Dubrowski in London. The term is widely used in the social and scientific literature and is in common, everyday usage. Yet, despite shared understanding of the word homophobia, there are some important limitations surrounding its use.

Homophobia as fear

George Weinberg first popularised the term homophobia in his (1972) book *Society and the Healthy Homosexual*. Its invention marked a watershed in lesbian and gay scholarship because it located the 'problem' of homosexuality, not in homosexuals, but in heterosexuals who were intolerant of lesbians and gay men (Herek, 2004). Homophobia is derived from the Greek word *phobia* meaning fear and it has come to conceptualise the fear of lesbians, gay men and bisexuals (LGB). Fear of having their own manhood questioned is believed to motivate heterosexual men's hostility towards gay men. A man's heterosexuality is proved, not in his relationship with a woman, but in his not being gay. (Some) heterosexual men, therefore, assert their heterosexuality by marking the separation between their own perceived status as 'real' men and that of gay men. While female heterosexuality *is* proved by a woman's relationship with a man, the threat of being called lesbian is used to intimidate (heterosexual and lesbian) women into female heteronormative appearance or behaviour. With its connotations of fear, homophobia inadequately characterises the hostility expressed towards homosexuals. Some would argue that anti-gay hostility is more consistent with anger – and its association with aggression – rather than fear (Herek, 2004); further, the emotions of disgust and repulsion are those which are most commonly articulated about lesbians and gay men (Valentine and McDonald, 2004).

Homophobia as a mental disorder

A phobia is a diagnostic category of mental disorder. Phobias are an irrational and persistent fear and they invite parallels with other forms of phobia – such as claustrophobia and agoraphobia. Being a lesbian or a gay man was considered a mental disorder in the *Diagnostic and Statistical Manual (DSM) II* and diagnostic labels such as neurosis, narcissism and nervous breakdown have frequently been applied to lesbians and gay men. The use of a term which implies psychiatric disorder continues the association between mental illness and homosexual identities. Similar arguments – since discredited – were developed to suggest that racism was a psychological disorder which left white people universally sick.

Moreover, if homophobes are mentally ill, the implication is that they should be treated with compassion and leniency (Kitzinger, 1996). Phobia as terminology, suggests that behaviour which is irrational and out of control is a 'normal' response to homosexuality. It makes possible a homosexual panic defence as a mitigating circumstance for murder. There have been cases in both the US and the UK where charges of murder of gay men have been reduced to manslaughter on these grounds.

Homophobia as an individual problem

Unlike sexism and racism, which were developed as political concepts in liberation movements, homophobia takes its origins in psychology (Kitzinger, 1996). Psychology locates the problem of homophobia in an individual's psychopathology and replaces political explanations with personal ones (Kitzinger, 1996). Writers from black and feminist perspectives have rejected the use of xenophobia (fear of strangers), misogyny (hatred of women) or gynophobia (fear of women) as inadequate to the task of conceptualising racism and sexism. The problem of locating anti-gay prejudice with individuals is that it is easy to dismiss homophobia as pertaining to the actions and behaviour of a small number of extreme people: it marks a separation between me and them (not homophobic vs. homophobic) – and *they* are usually seen as card carrying members of the British National Party. Black and feminist perspectives have also shown that personal forms of racism and sexism are often overemphasised at the expense of other institutional forms. The widespread use of race awareness training (RAT) in the 1980s was extensively critiqued because the focus on individuals ignored the material, social and political conditions that helped to reproduce discrimination and racist ideas (Solomos, 2003).

Internalised homophobia

Homophobia enables us to see the violence of 'queer bashing' and the bombing of the *Admiral Duncan* pub – these are violent acts perpetrated by others. But homophobia is also used to describe the internal or psychological state of lesbians and gay men. Internalised homophobia refers to the distress, lack of social support, maladaptive coping behaviours, greater alcohol consumption and low self-esteem experienced by some lesbians and gay men when they encounter hostility and rejection from heterosexuals. The term suggests that lesbians, gay men and bisexual people (LGB) fear or loathe themselves and it focuses attention on the psychological health of the victims of homophobia. Internalised homophobia suggests that a gay teenager who commits suicide, does so out of the same irrational fear that characterises the behaviour of those who have subjected her/him to bullying. Moreover, the term limits our understanding of the phenomenon. The poor mental health of lesbians and gay men may not be the result of internalised homophobia, but rather the consequence of living in a world which constructs them as inferior. To name suicide as a possible outcome of heterosexism shifts the focus of attention from blaming the victim to the social and political environment which allows the bullying of young lesbians and gay men to go unchecked and which privileges discourses of heteronormative masculinity and femininity.

Contradiction in (the) terms

Contrary to beliefs that it is a relatively new word, heterosexism first appeared as a parallel term to homophobia around the same time in 1972 (Herek, 2004); but its use is much less frequent. Its relation to the concept of homophobia is assumed to be simply a question of degree (Stewart, 1995). Homophobia is reserved for the most virulent and visible forms of anti-gay prejudice; it is often associated with some type of action. It is always intentional. Because of these connotations, there has been considerable resistance to the replacement of homophobia by another term. Opponents argue that alternative concepts – in particular heterosexism – diminish our rage or 'dull our pain' (Mohin in Kitzinger and Perkins, 1993: 60). Others are reluctant because the meaning of homophobia is widely understood (Rothblum and Bond, 1996). By contrast, heterosexism is often described in broad, vague terms and appears to be benign. It is frequently described as 'unintentional' (Gruskin, 1999); 'careless and unthinking' (Stewart, 1995); 'unconscious' (McFarlane, 1998); and is founded on errors of 'omission' or 'neglect' (Wilton, 2000). The characterisation of prejudice as something that is unintentional is usually made by those outside (rather than within) political movements. The McPherson report suggested that institutional racism in the Metropolitan Police – which led to the acquittal of those responsible for the murder of Stephen Lawrence – was unwitting. By constructing racism or heterosexism as unthinking, society is absolved from the responsibility of tackling them. Current understandings of heterosexism as unintentional have meant that even long-standing advocates of lesbian, gay and bisexual liberation believe the struggle against it is less significant.

As concepts, homophobia and heterosexism are profoundly contradictory. Paradoxically, while homophobia is primarily located in individuals, its effects are political. Because it gives name to our collective revulsion at acts of atrocities, it mobilises political opposition (in the form of demonstrations, lesbians' abseiling in the House of Lords, storming the BBC early evening news bulletin and protests by the pressure group *Outrage*). Heterosexism, which is structural and macro-level, invokes struggle using the 'meagre, individual resources of clothing, hairstyle and body language' (Wilton, 1997: 218). Its subtlety renders it difficult to define and hence to combat. Developing our understanding of anti-gay prejudice is limited by the fact that the terms are used as synonyms. In one of the few texts devoted to homophobia and heterosexism, their meanings overlap: both are defined as discrimination based on sexual orientation (Rothblum and Bond, 1996). Elsewhere, they are used interchangeably to mean discrimination and oppression. Learning some lessons from anti-racism suggests that discrimination and oppression refer to two different concepts and processes. Discrimination is rooted in the word to distinguish and refers to the unfair or unequal treatment of groups or individuals. It is evidenced in prejudicial behaviour against the interests of less powerful groups. Legislation is the key mechanism for dealing with discrimination (Dalrymple and Burke, 1995), but it is only able to target the most blatant forms. Yet, even in those instances where it is easiest to document and to prove, legislation to combat 'race' and sex discrimination has achieved relatively limited gains for black people and women. For example, despite the 1970 Equal Pay Act being on statute for more than 30 years, men still earn 17 per cent more than women working in similar jobs with equivalent skills and qualifications (retrieved 15 November 2005 from http://www.statistics.gov.uk). Moreover, sex and 'race' discrimination laws have frequently been used to redress inequalities experienced by men and white people.

Many people do not understand the term heterosexism, believing it to be prejudice against heterosexuals; others suggest that the term should be homosexism. While sexism refers to the privileging of men over women and racism refers to the privileging of white people over black people, heterosexism refers to the privileging of heterosexuality over homosexuality and its assumed normality. The term seeks to draw attention to the ways that heterosexuality is inscribed in institutions, cultural practices and everyday interactions.

The use of two terms is unhelpful because it implies they are two separate processes. It suggests that the violence or bullying described by homophobia is intentional (which it is undoubtedly is), but that assumptions about the superiority of heterosexuality are unconscious (which they should not be). Furthermore, the continued use of two terms interchangeably uncouples the overt manifestations of prejudice from the conceptual understandings of how such discrimination is perpetuated. Thus homophobia is reduced to a personal prejudice with no reference to the power and processes which sustain that prejudice: acts of discrimination are separated from theories of oppression. While homophobia is the most visible and direct form of discrimination, it is also the most exceptional. By focusing attention on the exceptional we ignore the everyday manifestations of oppression. Homophobia lacks explanation (other than individual prejudice); it can be eradicated by self-awareness, 'by learning the facts and by personal encounters with lesbians and gay men' (Ben-Ari, 2001: 121). Because of this, homophobia is limited in its ability to delineate the social, cultural, structural and institutional processes which serve to maintain the compulsory status of heterosexuality. By using the term homophobia, we see the goal only as the removal of discrimination, rather than a reinvention of the whole system.

The changing social landscape requires new conceptual understandings

The early twenty-first century has signalled a change in the social and political landscape for lesbians and gay men. Hitherto, discrimination against lesbians, gay men and bisexual people was explicitly sanctioned in legislation. Recent legislative changes mean that those mechanisms of the state which enforced discrimination have almost all been overturned. Furthermore, some legislation has been enacted to prevent discrimination (see Appendix A). For the first time, queer bashing is no longer seen as an inevitable consequence of being visibly homosexual, but has been recognised as a hate crime. Same-sex domestic abuse is acknowledged in the Domestic Violence, Crime and Victims Act 2004. There has been considerable progress in the area of legislative reform. Some commentators suggest that lesbian, gay and bisexual equality is now achieved; however, important though these gains are, they do not herald a battle won. The changing political context requires new understandings of the processes which maintain inequality; heterosexism is a theoretical concept that can help us to do this.

Towards a theory of heterosexism

Sexism, racism and disabilism are perpetuated in beliefs about the inherent inferiority of women, black people and disabled people. Similarly, heterosexism is based on assumptions about the inferiority of lesbians, gay men and bisexuals. Researchers have traditionally sought evidence to account for the difference of homosexuality; this difference is always constructed as inferior. The nature of homosexual inferiority has had a long history and has taken many forms.

Biological inferiority

The body was believed to show evidence of differences between homosexuals and 'normal' heterosexuals in skull dimensions, postures, gestures and mannerisms. Researchers sought markers of deviance in lesbian bodies; they claimed that the typical lesbian had different genitals to heterosexual women and these differences were pathological (Terry, 1995). More recently, LeVay (1993) claimed to have discovered the 'gay brain': in particular, the hypothalamus in gay men was said to be smaller than in heterosexual men. (Smaller brain size was also related to 'race' and gender in the late nineteenth century.) Research has also suggested that lesbians have different hearing abilities and finger length ratios to heterosexual women (Birke, 2002).

Hormonal imbalance

The notion of homosexuals as a third sex dominated early twentieth-century constructions of the causes of homosexuality. Homosexuality was an intermediate sex and homosexuals were said to be stuck at a primitive stage of evolutionary development; they were 'unfinished specimens . . . a status they shared with savages and criminals' (Terry, 1995: 135). The subsequent discovery of sex hormones lent support to this theory; male and female sex hormones (testosterone and oestrogen) are believed to be imbalanced in lesbians and gay men. Lesbians are said to be mannish and gay men effeminate.

Genetic inferiority

Some have suggested that male homosexuality may be a result of genetic abnormality: gay men (it is said) tend to be born of elderly mothers. The late 1990s saw an increase in genetic explanations for homosexuality: some claimed to have found patterns of homosexuality in studies of twins, while others are said to have identified the 'gay gene'. Locating a gene raises the problem of testing the foetus in the womb and possible subsequent abortion (Birke, 2002).

Psychological inferiority

Lesbians and gay men are said to be aggressive, masochistic, destructive, deceitful, neurotic, obsessive, narcissistic, paranoid and psychotic. Being a lesbian or gay man was a mental disorder in the *DSM II*.

Moral inferiority

Lesbians and gay men have been considered to be responsible for the rise in crime, murder, racism, societal chaos, and weakening of the family.

Their ascribed immorality means they are less trustworthy and more likely to be a threat to the state.

Emotional inferiority

Lesbians and gay men are said to be incapable of sustaining an emotional relationship with a partner. Their relationships are co-dependent (lesbians' tendency to merge) and seldom satisfying. They are emotionally immature, have irrational attractions and are deeply lonely.

Inferior upbringing

The lack of normal childhood relations with their parents is said to cause homosexuality. The combination of an over-intense relationship with the mother and an unsatisfactory relationship with a weak father has been said to be typical for homosexual men. Lesbians are the result of an emotionally disturbed childhood; lesbians are said to hate and reject both parents (Bene, 1965a, 1965b).

Sexual inferiority

Gay men, in particular, are said to be promiscuous and have unnatural desires and sexual practices. They are said to pose a threat to children and young people. Lesbians are said to be asexual.

These theories of inferiority act as pre-existing frameworks of meaning around homosexuality and serve to oppress lesbians, gay men and bisexuals. Heterosexism is the term used to describe this oppression; oppression implies agency; it moulds, restrains and restricts (Frye, 1998). Celia Kitzinger (1996) provides an illustration:

> . . . when there is *no* anti-lesbian explosion from your parents because you have de-dyked your house before their visit; when there is no queer-bashing after an evening's clubbing, because you anticipated trouble and booked a taxi home; when you are not dismissed from work, because you stayed in the closet; when you are not subjected to prurient questions because you have talked about your partner euphemistically as a friend – when these non-events slip by as part of many gay men and lesbians' daily routine, has *nothing* really happened? Rather, heterosexism has been functioning in its most effective and most deadly way. In an oppressive society, it is not necessary, most of the time, to beat us up, to murder or torture us to ensure our silence and invisibility. This is because a climate of terror has been created instead in which most gay people *voluntarily* and of our own free will

choose to remain silent and invisible. (Kitzinger, 1996: 11, emphasis in original)

The example shows the pervasiveness of heterosexism; it functions by circumscribing opportunities and prescribing certain kinds of behaviour. It is characterised by an absence – where it appears that nothing has really happened. Oppression imposes a particular world-view which permeates the social and political fabric of our lives; it enforces silence and invisibility. Heterosexist beliefs not only enforce certain kinds of behaviour, but they also justify exclusion from social resources, such as housing, employment, education, health and social care. This system of beliefs together with the values, cultural norms, language, institutional practices and structures are the means by which relations of domination and subordination are asserted. Getting rid of heterosexuality as an institution means a complete overhaul of the system:

(It means) getting rid of sexual difference. It also means abolishing most of the legal system, marriage, the family, most cultural and national traditions, the church, in all its forms, all sects, and most aspects of all other religions too, the tax system, work patterns, childcare arrangements, the distribution of wealth. It means rethinking the language, rebuilding our houses, remaking most of the sculptures, repainting the pictures and rewriting the books. (Duncker, 1993: 148)

Our individual relationships and our social organisations are established in such a way as to assume, and thereby privilege, heterosexuality. This coercion has been conceived as 'you-will-be-straight-or-you-will-not-be' (Wittig, 1988); that is, 'compulsory heterosexuality' (Rich, 1983) does not allow an equal alternative. As Warner contends (1993) western culture insists that humanity and heterosexuality are synonymous. Beliefs about the superiority of heterosexuality (in values, discourse and culture) together with discriminatory practices (in institutions, resources and services) and attitudes (assumptions, stereotypes and prejudices) work together to perpetuate the oppression of lesbians, gay men and bisexual people.

In the rest of the chapter, I aim to develop an understanding of heterosexism as a theory of lesbian, gay and bisexual oppression. It is intended, not as a definitive version, but instead to stimulate debate and to explore the ways we can begin to make the invisible, visible, the silent, spoken and to reveal the dichotomised power relationship in the homosexual/heterosexual binary. While there is agreement that there are some commonalities in the processes which maintain social divisions (Dominelli,

2002), it is less clear how these are manifested. Sexism and racism are well theorised by comparison to heterosexism; by drawing some parallels with them, it may be possible to uncover some of the ways heterosexism operates. Heterosexism is not monolithic, but is constantly shifting and contextual; it exists in a multiplicity of sites. Some of the processes by which it is perpetuated are analysed below and include privilege; the routine presumption of heterosexuality; the public/private divide; the silencing of sexual identities; 'just the same' arguments; reverse discrimination; language and discourse; and the moral backlash.

Privilege

Privilege is a characteristic of oppression; it confers advantage for one group over another. By its favoured status, privilege grants access to social, cultural, moral, linguistic and political resources. Those who possess privilege are often unable, or unwilling, to acknowledge it. Men (as a group) cannot see how they benefit from sexism; whites cannot comprehend how they gain privilege from racism; nor can the non-disabled see how they accrue advantage from disablism. Privilege is an invisible package of unearned assets which can be cashed in daily:

> (It) is like an invisible, weightless knapsack of special provisions, maps, passports, codebooks, visas, clothes, tools and blank checks. (McIntosh, 1998: 165)

It works most effectively when it is taken for granted; those who hold privileged status see it as natural, normative, average, unthinking, morally neutral and also ideal. For example, heterosexuality is the preferred living arrangement in which to bring up children. Because the family is seen to be morally neutral, and children are believed to fare better where there are two opposite-sexed parents, heterosexuality is construed as ideal. It is taken for granted that heterosexuality is superior to homosexuality and there are abundant examples in legislation, social policy and in our wider social arrangements. In attempting to understand the ways in which she enjoyed unearned 'white' privilege, McIntosh (1998) documents the daily conditions that white people take for granted. A similar exercise, by drawing on her examples, helps to uncover some of the privileges accruing to heterosexuality:

1. When I meet someone for the first time, I do not need to consider whether or not to disclose my heterosexuality.
2. If I choose to disclose my heterosexuality, people will not interpret this as a sexual advance.

3. I can if I wish arrange to be in the company of people of my sexual identity most of the time.
4. I can be almost certain that if I move house my neighbours will be neutral or pleasant towards me.
5. As a student, I can be sure that curricula materials will present my heterosexuality positively.
6. The media can represent someone of my sexual identity perform an act of intimacy (such as kissing) without this being considered remarkable.
7. As a member of a religious organisation, there is no contradiction between my heterosexuality and my faith.
8. My children will not be taunted or bullied because of my heterosexuality.
9. I am not considered biased on account of my heterosexuality.
10. I can automatically count on the support and understanding of my family and friends when I disclose problems in my heterosexual relationship.
11. As a teenager, my heterosexuality will not be dismissed as something I will grow out of by people close to me.
12. My heterosexuality is not universally considered a threat to (or a negative influence upon) children.
13. My partner will not be euphemistically referred to as my 'best friend', long-time companion or entirely ignored.
14. People do not generally assume that my primary heterosexual relationship will be short-lived.

Privilege is a mechanism which asserts the superiority of heterosexuality. Because privilege is unacknowledged and unreflective (it rarely has need to be), it allows those who hold it the power to deny or ignore the privilege they hold. This base of unacknowledged privilege is not only unconscious; members of privileged groups have been conditioned into oblivion about its existence (McIntosh, 1998). Heterosexuality protects from many kinds of hostility, distress, moral judgements and violence. Privilege then, confers belonging with people around us and it is a means of making social systems work for those who hold it. The privileged status of marriage as a heterosexual institution is continued in the new legislation which grants same-sex couples the right to register their partnerships, while the social status conferred by marriage is reserved for opposite-sex couples. Moreover, the social privilege of heterosexuality is confirmed by the unequal status of LGB citizenship.

The routine presumption of heterosexuality

Heterosexism is also defined as the routine presumption of heterosexuality. This is subtly different to the way in which sexism is maintained. While male experience is normative and has often accounted for both male and female experience, women are not universally presumed to be men. Similarly, on a conceptual level, heterosexual experience encompasses homosexual experience. For example, women's health is often believed to account for the health of both heterosexual and lesbian women (see Chapter 8). But the heterosexual presumption also operates in everyday lives. On first meeting, a person is assumed to be heterosexual unless they identify themselves otherwise. This information is not usually volunteered; heterosexuals do not go round saying 'hello, I'm heterosexual' because there is no need to do so (Peel, 2001: 549). One of the many ways that heterosexuality is maintained is that it rarely has to attest to its existence.

Many heterosexuals, then, do not think about their heterosexuality except as an unquestioned given or as a personal choice which has no effect on the rest of their lives or on the lives of others. Heterosexual (like male, 'white' and ablebodied) is always implicit and unspoken. When Kitzinger and Wilkinson (1993) produced a special issue of *Feminism & Psychology* on the topic of heterosexuality, they posed the question in their call for papers: 'How does your heterosexuality contribute to your feminist politics?' It was met with responses ranging from blank incomprehension to anger. The invitation positioned potential contributors as heterosexual; it seems that until then, many had considered themselves to be generic women. One woman, despite having lived monogamously with a man for 26 years, seemed to be unable to identify herself as heterosexual. Others (who had talked freely of their husbands and had never spoken on lesbian issues) wrote angrily: 'How dare you assume I'm heterosexual?' and 'Don't you think you are making one hell of an assumption?' (1993: 5). Kitzinger and Wilkinson (1993) had made explicit an assumption that the (heterosexual) women had allowed to be implicit in their everyday lives. Their unwillingness to accept the label heterosexual suggests that they were unable to acknowledge the privilege which their heterosexuality had hitherto afforded them.

One of the most ubiquitous features of the world as experienced by oppressed people is the double bind – 'situations in which options are reduced to a very few and all of them expose one to penalty, censure or deprivation' (Frye, 1998: 147). The double bind maintains the privileged status of heterosexuality by imposing contradictory constraints on LGB people. In the previous example, lesbians made visible the heterosexuality of heterosexual women. One might assume then, that heterosexual women would be comfortable with an assumption that they were lesbian. This is not always the case. When I 'came out' in a sexuality workshop, my co-convenor came out as heterosexual (even though I had previously discussed my disclosure with her), presumably because she did not want to be mistaken for a lesbian. In discussion in *Challenging Heterosexism* workshops, many participants have failed to see this as an example of heterosexism. Instead, they suggest that the trainer may have intended to be helpful in giving information about herself. (This assumes that the information is neutral.) I wonder whether my co-convenor would have come out as heterosexual if I had not first come out as lesbian. It would seem not. Her heterosexuality would have been taken for granted, my sexual identity would have been wrongly assumed. There are numerous examples of heterosexual celebrities distancing themselves from any suggestion of homosexuality. A number have taken court action or placed notices in newspapers to assert their heterosexuality. The recent spate of heterosexual actors playing LGBT roles is a further example: while it is now a safe career move for straight actors to take on gay roles, most have been at pains to distance themselves from any suggestion of themselves being gay. The actors were so 'extraordinarily' heterosexual: one was cast alongside his (off-screen) opposite sex partner to provide a sexual alibi (Hensher, 2005: 22). Coming out then, is not the equivalent experience for heterosexuals and homosexuals:

> It may be easy to understand why it might be offensive to treat heterosexuals as if they were gay, but less easy to recognise why it might be equally offensive to treat lesbians and gay men as if they were heterosexual. (Wilton, 1999: 7)

It is offensive to treat LGB as if they were heterosexual because it erases their existence – it is only possible to erase heterosexuality temporarily or situationally. The risks and perils about coming out as heterosexual are not the same as coming out as homosexual. Heterosexuals are not 'straight-bashed' because they are heterosexual. Compulsory heterosexuality means that heterosexuals may resist being positioned either as heterosexual or homosexual.

Decisions about disclosure are also a double bind: disclosure is said to be flaunting oneself, while non-disclosure is deceitful. Coming out is at once compulsory and forbidden as Eve Kosofsky-Sedgwick illustrates in an example of a teacher who was dismissed from his post. In a first court action, he was judged to have disclosed too much about his sexual identity;

but on appeal, he was deemed to have not disclosed enough (cf. Kosofsky-Sedgwick, 1993). The suggestion that coming out as heterosexual and coming out as LGB is a parallel process ignores the routine presumption of heterosexuality.

The public/private divide in the lives of lesbians, gay men and bisexuals

The public sphere is overwhelmingly heterosexual (Richardson, 1996, 2000). Our public institutions – the criminal justice system, medicine, education, the media, public services and religion – are founded on the concepts of heterosexuality; heterosexuality is everywhere assumed in social life. By contrast, the notion that homosexuality is something which is conducted in private has been regulated through legislation. Between 1885 and 1967 in the UK, all male homosexual acts whether committed in public or private were illegal (Weeks, 1979). The 1967 Sexual Offences Act is widely believed to have liberalised the laws on male homosexuality, but it did so on condition that lesbians, gay men and bisexuals not only conducted their relationships in private, but also lived their homosexuality in private. The Earl of Arran, one of the bill's supporters, declared that 'any form of ostentatious behaviour . . . any public flaunting would be utterly distasteful and would make the sponsors of the bill regret what they have done' (Simpson, 1994: 265). Following the introduction of the legislation, the penalties for public displays of homosexuality were strengthened. The number of convictions for homosexual offences increased (despite the apparent liberalisation) and the police were engaged in the active surveillance of lesbian, gay and bisexual meeting places (Weeks, 1979). Decades later, privacy framed political discourses surrounding the repeal of the age of consent, and previously, in constructing arguments for the introduction of section 28 (Waites, 2003). The Shadow Home Secretary, Anne Widdicombe, argued that 'what people do in private is their own business' and Margaret Thatcher, the then Prime Minister, apparently did not object to homosexuals *per se*, but disliked them in publicly visible groups. The meanings of privacy were extremely limited: a hotel room was not private, nor was a house with a third person in it if the bedroom doors were not locked. The exhortation to privacy has not, however, reliably offered protection to gay men. In the US 1986 *Bowers v. Hardwick* decision, the Supreme Court judgement denied a gay man the right to engage in consensual sex with another man in the privacy of his own bedroom. But privacy does not relate only to sexual behaviour: the term 'flaunting' suggests that all visible LGB identity should be toned down. Heterosexuals are offended by LGB 'show'.

Lesbians, gay men and bisexuals did not choose the closet; they were forced into it.

But while privacy is not simply a personal choice that lesbians and gay men make, it allows them to deflect unwanted attention about their sexual identity. Labour politicians, speaking in support of gay colleagues who had come out or who were outed by the press, avoided further discussion by arguing that it was a private issue. Conservative politicians, who have publicly opposed the civil rights of lesbians and gay men, have also used privacy to police the boundaries of what may be discussed. The family of Mary Cheney, the daughter of Bush's vice-presidential running-mate, avoided questions about her sexuality by claiming that it was a private matter (Johnson, 2002). Privacy is successfully used in liberal discourses, by lesbians, gay men and bisexuals, to avoid unwanted intrusions into their lives. The argument is often made: my personal life is my business and not anyone else's. The notion of privacy is also used as a damage limitation strategy. A trade union, seeking to dispel the myth that gay men are paedophiles, made the following argument in a booklet about gay rights and fighting prejudice:

> A homosexual person is no more likely than a heterosexual person to make sexual advances to clients, customers, fellow workers or the general public . . . Gay workers have the same physical, mental and emotional characteristics as heterosexuals . . . They only differ in being gay. That might have implications for their private lives but ought to make no difference to their working lives. (cited in Thompson, 1997: 137)

Rather than tackle the offensiveness of the assumption that gay men are a threat to children, the argument turns to the 1967 legislation, that same-sex behaviour is only performed in private. A clear separation is maintained between a private life, where sexuality may be expressed, and a public, working life, where sexual behaviour is taboo. The suggestion that gay men regard children as valid objects of sexual desire is circumvented, rather than actively confronted. The boundary is used to draw a demarcation line between the public and the private, and, in this instance, allows some limited protection for gay men without challenging the underlying assumptions.

While lesbians and gay men are exhorted to keep their lives private, the quintessential domain of privacy – the family – has long been denied them. LGB have often lost child custody cases, were unable to access fertilisation services and were barred from jointly adopting children. Section

28 determined that same-sex families were inferior because they were only *pretended* family relationships rather than real ones. Heterosexism then, allows only a certain form of private life for lesbians, gay men and bisexuals: they are entitled to a circumscribed existence on condition that they do not seek full membership in society. When sexual minorities accept that their private lives (i.e. their identities as lesbians, bisexuals and gay men) do not form part of everyday interactions (as those of heterosexual identities do), they are agreeing to a second-class stake in social life. In the 1980s, feminists sought to politicise the personal, to draw attention to the political and social basis of women's oppression. The domestic, personal sphere was not seen to lie outside of social and political life, but to be fundamentally interwoven with it. The sphere occupied by lesbians, gay men and bisexuals is not the personal and domestic arena, however, but a private one. The connotations of privacy imply an arena that is not generally known, a confidential space that is peculiar to oneself. What is private is not, and should not, be open to public gaze. Lesbians, gay men and bisexuals need to politicise the private.

Politicians commonly cite the private nature of homosexuality as a reason for denying civil rights to lesbian, gay and bisexual people: because it is a personal matter it does not warrant political intervention in the form of enabling social policies. This has a number of implications for lesbian and gay citizenship. Because their identities properly 'belong' in the private sphere, lesbians and gay men have no basis on which to present themselves in public institutions: in hospitals, schools, to the police or social services. An equal citizenship does not seek the right to do what one wants to in private, but is concerned with establishing public lesbian, gay and bisexual identities. The right to a private life is enshrined in human rights legislation; what lesbians, gay men and bisexuals lack, is the right to a public life.

The silencing of sexual identity

Oscar Wilde famously described homosexuality as 'the love that dare not speak its name'. The silencing of sexual identity is often taken to indicate an absence; Rosenblum (1996) argues that instead it signifies the presence of a multitude of barriers; silence and invisibility are themselves human rights violations. Injunctions to silence are maintained in everyday conversation. Any mention of one's sexual identity may be met with accusations of: 'ramming it down people's throats', 'being blatant', 'flaunting it'; even the language of disclosure suggests the secretive (e.g. confiding), sinful or criminal (e.g. confessing) quality in being open about one's gay identity. Heterosexism then is discursively produced by a conspiracy of silence (Blumenfeld, 1992: 6).

In their research about the social positioning of sexual identity in the workplace, Ward and Winstanley (2003) point to the multi-faceted nature of silence: as absence of response, as a form of suppression and censorship and as self-protection and resistance. Even in apparently forward-thinking organisations with progressive diversity management practices, silence was a significant theme:

> The reaction to my coming out was no reaction. I didn't encounter any hostility . . . The big difference I noticed in the way colleagues treat me is the degree of interest they show in my life outside work. When I was married, it was a two-way process; there was mutual interest in the mundane things in life, what we did at the weekend, kids, pets, even the trip to the supermarket. That way of communicating is now closed off to me to some extent. I've noticed that I can be asking people about what they do, but as soon as I start talking about what I'm doing they shut down, because they are not prepared to hear . . . (Ward and Winstanley, 2003: 1266)

By avoiding this social interaction, colleagues in the workplace clearly marked out the boundaries of what could be talked about and what must be left unsaid. Talk about everyday events with people around us gives meaning to them and provides a social connection with others; it often acts to mitigate some of the impersonal effects of work (Ward and Winstanley, 2003). While homosexuality is silenced, heterosexuality is silent. Many heterosexuals appear to believe they live in a sexually neutral world, rather than one in which heterosexuality is dominant. Lesbians, gay men and bisexuals are considered to have a sexual orientation, while heterosexuals do not. This is illustrated in the treatment of a gay man who was working in the government department responsible for the repeal of section 28. He was moved from his job, ostensibly because his managers thought it was inappropriate for a gay man to have a say in the repeal of the legislation: by virtue of being a gay man he could not be impartial (Ward and Winstanley, 2003).

Heterosexuality as a silent term has implications beyond the identities of individuals. Assumptions of heterosexuality so permeate our daily lives, that many heterosexuals simply cannot hear or see heterosexism. In a response to the first *BMJ* editorial about lesbian and bisexual women's health needs, Julietta Patnick (the Programme Director) stated that the

NHS Cervical Screening Programme (CSP) offers screening to all women without enquiring about their sexual behaviour (Patnick and Davidson, 2003, retrieved 5 November 2003 from http://bmjournals.com/cgi/letters/327/7421/939). I encountered many similar claims from heterosexual women in audiences when I gave conference papers about lesbians' experiences of smear tests. Perhaps the reasons that lesbians 'hear' the question about their sexual identity and heterosexual women do not, can be accounted for by their different positions within the CSP. Simply, heterosexual women may not recognise the question 'what contraception do you use?' as an implicit question about their sexual identity. (Lesbians, mostly, do not need to control their fertility because sex is not linked to reproduction.) Sometimes, health professionals ask: 'Do you think you might be pregnant?' because they assume that (presumed) heterosexual women become pregnant accidentally and communicate this assumption during the smear test. (Lesbian pregnancies are more likely to be planned than accidental.) Heterosexual women may also fail to hear a question 'when did you last have sexual intercourse?' as problematic. Most lesbians would need to consider whether their sexual behaviour 'counted' as sexual intercourse because the term usually refers to penis-in-the-vagina sex. In addition, heterosexuality is assumed, not only in the individual interaction with a health care professional, but throughout the screening programme. Heterosexuality is inscribed in health promotion materials, the size of the speculum, the term 'family planning' and the heterosexualised nature of the smear itself (its classic missionary position). (For further discussion about heterosexism in cervical screening see Chapter 7.)

Why can't homosexuals be just like heterosexuals?

Oppression operates through assumptions of a deficit and it demands that those deemed inferior approximate the characteristics of the superior group. The price of acceptance is to become what your oppressor wants you to be: just like them. Anti-racist analyses delineate similar processes of accommodation in which black people are expected to assimilate to white cultural norms: by wearing western clothes (not the *hijab*), eating western foods and by adopting Eurocentric traditions, values and ways of thinking. Women have often been excluded from public institutions, such as law schools and military colleges in the US, on the basis that intellectually and physically they were different from and inferior to men. Feminists successfully used the argument – that women are just the same as men – to secure access to public institutions from which they had been previously debarred. But while physical access has been secured to some elite establishments, the terms of that access have been highly circumscribed. Fine and Addelston (1996) argue that access has been granted disproportionately to upper and middle class white women; but their presence has not changed the structure of institutions. Once inside these institutions – that now represent themselves as diverse – the women came to express attitudes, beliefs and experiences that mimicked those of men. The conceptual framework of sameness and difference determines the basis of acceptance. Being just like the dominant group means that minorities lose their distinct identities. Being different constructs minorities as inferior.

Just the same arguments are not only used by mainstream society, but also by oppressed groups. Common strategies of those seeking acceptance and tolerance are to emphasise the similarities between themselves and those of the dominant group. Such normalising strategies have been used to argue that lesbian and gay parenting is indistinguishable from heterosexual parenting: LGB parents help children with their homework, make packed lunches and argue about bedtimes (Clarke, 2001). Because *family* is a heterosexual concept (lesbians and gay men have only had *pretend* families), lesbians and gay men who want to be considered a family (or to adopt a family) must approximate heterosexuality. Rather than posing a challenge to the family as a heterosexual institution – for example, an analysis that argued the benefits of having two same-sex parents on conceptions about the sexual division of labour – many of the debates have instead served to bolster traditional family forms. Thus LGB who most conform to the values, beliefs, behaviours and lives of heterosexuals will be those most likely to be accepted by society. Heterosexism, then, determines the nature of social and political participation and sets the terms of debate. Assimilation irons out the differences between homosexuality and heterosexuality; but it does so by imposing the standards of heterosexuality (these arguments are developed in Chapter 9).

Reverse discrimination

The statement that homosexuals are oppressed is often met with the claim that heterosexuals are oppressed too: it is a means of discounting heterosexism. Such claims have led one theorist to coin the phrase 'the problem of the oppressed heterosexual' (Brickell, 2001: 225). The links with sexism and racism are important because one invidious ideological backlash has been the notion of *political correctness*. The accusation of being *PC* suggests that the person pointing out oppression is taking things too far. It claims that being female is given preference over being male and blackness is unconditionally valued over whiteness.

Privilege rests on the assumption that there are no power differentials between one group and another; as a consequence, homosexuals and heterosexuals are believed to enjoy the same access to social, cultural and institutional resources. It operates by making a false equivalence. If equality is already achieved, then any (minority) group which receives different treatment is seen (by the majority) to be granted special rights as the following example illustrates.

The Ministry of Women's Affairs in Wellington, New Zealand hosted a catered meeting for lesbians who work in the civil service (for a full discussion of this incident see Brickell, 2001). This meeting, which came to be known as the lesbian lunch, was widely reported in the news media under such headlines as 'Government to give lesbians a free lunch'. One of the daily newspapers encouraged readers to express their views in the letters page: readers wrote to demand that men also wanted lunch laid on. Another suggested that some women employees came out of the closet when they heard that a free lunch was available. In their reports, newspapers frequently compared lesbians with other occupational groups with the apparent intention of making lesbians seem ridiculous:

> There are some weird and wonderful collectives in this world. One of the more unusual in our experience is the Canadian Association of Seed Crushers, though the British Society of Deep Fat Fryers would run it close. So there should be no surprise that the Ministry of Women's Affairs has found another one. Lesbians working in government. (Brickell, 2001: 219–20)

The comparisons are interesting: *Seed Crushers* suggests a little known, and of equally little interest, trade association. *Deep Fat Fryers* connotes mundane kitchen skills. There is nothing discriminatory in the terms themselves, but they convey an offensive suggestion of triviality. Humour, or more precisely, ridicule, is an effective weapon in undermining claims to minority status. Similar mechanisms operated in relation to descriptions of feminists in the 1980s as bra-burning women's libbers. There is no recognition in these reports that lesbians are located in particular ways within workplace hierarchies, or that there may be difficulties in making contact with, or being visible to, other lesbians. Their needs for associating with others are posited as no different from those of a society of deep fat fryers. The media report is effective because it constructs a false equivalence between a minority interest trade association and lesbians as a minority group.

Some of the debates around the introduction of the civil partnership legislation rested on similar concepts. Unmarried heterosexuals claimed that they were also oppressed because their partners would not receive their pensions on their death (Peel, 2001). Their argument wilfully ignores the fact that heterosexual couples can make a choice to marry; civil partnerships offer second-class status and the privileged institution of marriage is reserved for heterosexuals. Any attempt to redress the balance of structured inequalities is undermined by notions of equality of opportunity. The concept of equal opportunity is profoundly individualistic and liberal: it assumes an individual will achieve the same educational success (for example), if everyone is treated as if they are the same. Those who claim reverse discrimination invoke such arguments as: heterosexuals are not singled out for special treatment so why should homosexuals be? Heterosexism is perpetuated by beliefs that we occupy a level playing-field. It confuses equality of opportunity with equality of outcome.

Language and discourse

Critical social theorists have drawn attention to the ways language is used in perpetuating oppression. For instance, 'he' as a generic pronoun was used to refer to both men and women. In the mid-1980s, the debate focused on terminology: language was seen to both reflect and reinforce power relations. These concerns were subsequently adopted as guidelines on anti-sexist, anti-racist and anti-disablist language in organisations such as the British Sociological Association (BSA). There was relatively little work on anti-heterosexist language. From the early 1990s, there has been a move within discursive psychology to consider the ways that discourse (all textual and spoken language) constructs oppression. Blatant comments are becoming increasingly less common. Instead, opponents of LGB rights draw on discourses which construct LGB people as inferior and make claims by association. For example, in Clarke's (1999) research an audience member in *Kilroy* undermines LGB's claims to provide good enough parenting:

> For a child to grow up, a child learns from parents okay, and for a child when – when they see loving relationships, it's normal for a child to see a man and a woman being loving with each other, it isn't normal (I bet a lot) will agree, it isn't normal [. . .] for a child to walk in a bedroom and see two men kissing each other on a bed, or two women kissing on a bed, it isn't a normal thing for a child to grow up with. (1999: 10)

This argument would not usually be described as discriminatory. But it is constructed in such a way that it functions to perpetuate heterosexism.

The speaker infers that LGB relationships are detrimental to a child's development by drawing on notions of homosexual recruitment: in witnessing homosexual relationships, the child will become LGB. The argument implies that LGB are abnormal, although it does not do so explicitly. (Indeed, some heterosexuals do not appear to think it *is* offensive to describe homosexuals as abnormal.) The speaker also suggests that only heterosexual relationships are loving relationships; in the extract, these are decontextualised as 'being loving'. Homosexual relationships, by contrast, are sexualised – they take place in the bedroom; they involve kissing; and there is no mention of love. All this is achieved indirectly and by implication. It is only possible because it draws upon existing heteronormative discourses.

Discursive psychological studies of racism and sexism have highlighted the way in which concerns about being heard as speaking from a prejudiced position are managed by speakers by constructing evaluations as mere factual descriptions. Participants employ a range of strategies which enable them to express remarks – such as he was a complete poof – that otherwise would be considered offensive. Speer and Potter (2000) note a dual concern to express a view and also manage it in a way that portrays the speaker as caring and egalitarian. In response to a question about his perceptions of a gay club, Ben (a heterosexual research participant) has to negotiate a line between lack of enjoyment which might indicate psychological trouble with gay people, with that of enjoyment which might suggest that Ben is gay or harbours gay feelings. His denials, mis-starts, frequent pauses, hesitation and self-repair indicate his dilemma. Awareness of heterosexism allows us to become attuned to the particular nuances of prejudiced talk.

The moral backlash

Unlike race, disability and gender, homosexuality has been centrally defined by discourses of morality (Warner, 1993). Feminism's insistence that men should share responsibility for child-rearing and domestic labour also met with a powerful right-wing backlash with links to fundamentalist Christianity (Bacchi, 1990). However, social conservatives have overwhelmingly seen LGB civil rights claims as a threat to the heterosexual family and traditional values. Proposals surrounding adoption, civil partnerships and the age of consent are said to contravene immutable human truths.

Right-wing strategists have frequently used homosexuality to divert attention from current social problems. George W. Bush's 2004 presidential campaign was a calculated (and successful) attempt to mobilise the

Republican vote by appealing to evangelical Christians through a ballot measure to ban gay marriage. In the eleven states where the ballot was being polled, tens of thousands of new voters were registered. Bush constituted same-sex marriage as the most important threat to the USA during a presidency in which he had waged an illegal war in Iraq, detained prisoners without trial in Guantanamo Bay and had overseen a period of increased economic disparity between the wealthy and the poor. Republicans achieved the Reagan landslide in 1980 using similar tactics.

Lesbians and gay men have become targets for persecution as a means of diverting attention away from other social ills such as economic recession, social upheaval or war. They have, at times, been constituted as posing a social danger to national security because of their supposed moral deviance. During the McCarthy era in the 1950s, homosexuals were routinely sacked from their jobs and imprisoned because they were seen to have less integrity, be susceptible to 'blackmail' and lacking in moral fibre (Faderman, 1992). The legacy of this period has been to create discursive practices which link homosexuality with immorality, disease, decadence and chaos. Subsequently, New Right ideology has drawn upon these discourses and blamed homosexuals for the alleged inability of the US to stand up to the Russians (Rubin, 1993). In the hysteria surrounding the HIV/AIDS pandemic, the so-called 'moral majority' claimed that diseased homosexuals would infect the entire nation and destroy the US (Shilts, 1987). In 2003, the Egyptian government created a moral panic about homosexuality through arbitrary arrest, imprisonment and the subsequent *Queen Boat* trials as a means of diverting attention from the country's economic recession (de Gruchy and Fish, 2004).

It may seem surprising in an increasingly secular age that arguments about religion and morality are used to invoke opposition to lesbian, gay and bisexual rights and continue to hold such sway. Moreover, they are returned to (in US elections in 1980 and 2004) and reformulated: they enabled, for example, the aspiring EU Commissioner, Rocco Buttiglione to suggest that homosexuality is a sin. Baroness Young and Brian Souter drew on similar arguments in the opposition to the lowering of the age of consent and the repeal of section 28. The arguments of the New Right have shifted to a more complex terrain with parameters which clearly define the inferior status of homosexuality (Waites, 2000). The church as an institution actively constructs homosexuality as inferior as seen in recent debates about whether Anglican priests can register their civil partnerships and remain a member of the clergy. If a priest wishes to register a partnership this might imply that the relationship is sexual; while the church allows its clergy to be non-practising homosexuals it does not accord them a sexual relationship. The ban rests on assumptions that gay sex is intrinsically more reprehensible than straight sex.

These are not the random utterances of a few, isolated individuals which may be disregarded as homophobic. Instead they draw upon a set of beliefs, ideological positions and institutional practices that have been sanctioned by religion, medicine, the law and culture and which specify the nature of homosexual inferiority. Homosexuals are inherently threatening: to institutional heterosexuality, to children, to family life, to morality. Those who use religious and moral arguments claim a higher ground (god is on our side); because of its place in cultural and social life, religious and moral arguments are accorded higher status than secular and rights-based arguments.

Conclusion

Although there have been numerous calls to replace homophobia with the term heterosexism, there has also been considerable resistance. This is partly because an (apparently) politicised term would be replaced by one that suggests that LGB oppression is unconscious. It is also because political activity, so far, has been directed to the removal of the most blatant forms of discrimination. Before the term homophobia can be superseded (it is not merely substitution), we need first to understand heterosexism as a theoretical concept, to recognise its similarities and differences to other forms of oppression and to analyse how it is perpetuated. Heterosexism may be commonplace, but it is neither mundane nor benign. Examples of it, however, are often benign and include the assumptions of heterosexuality implicit in employment application forms; assessment forms in social work; and sexual history taking in health care. In drawing parallels with other forms of oppression, the chapter has attempted to reveal how heterosexism is organised, for example, by making implicit privilege, explicit. There are also other parallels including assimilation (just the same arguments), the double bind, false equivalence and the construction of LGB issues (as with sexism) as private or personal concerns. By examining the processes which perpetuate the inferiority of homosexuality and the heterosexual assumption, the chapter has aimed to show that these can be seen, not simply as indications of homophobia, but as the mechanisms by which heterosexism is maintained.

The rest of the book is organised in two parts in order to analyse heterosexism in concrete situations. The first part deals with overarching themes and in doing so, draws on existing research to examine the pervasiveness of heterosexism in relation to access to health and social care (Chapter 2). Chapter 3 recognises that 'race', transgender, class, disability, bisexuality, geographic location and sexual identity are not occupied as separate and divisible aspects of the self, but as multiple identities. It considers the particular manifestations of heterosexism in relation to different LGBT identities. Chapter 4 investigates the ways in which research is constrained by heterosexist concepts. The invisibility of LGB populations is considered in Chapter 5 which discusses what is known about the demographic characteristics of the LGB population.

The second part of the book takes quantitative and qualitative data as case studies from a large UK research project of lesbian health to look specifically at the ways in which health and health care are permeated by heterosexism. Disclosure is a constant theme in lesbian, gay and bisexual health and social care research; Chapter 6 considers the ways in which lesbians negotiate disclosure and non-disclosure in their interactions with health professionals. They choose active and passive strategies of disclosure and non-disclosure. In Chapter 7, the positive and adverse experiences which lesbians report in their health care interactions with service providers are examined. Chapter 8 considers how current understandings about risk are constrained by heterosexism. The final chapter looks forward to new directions in equality agendas and to the opportunities and threats posed by policies of social inclusion and the establishment of a single equality commission.

2
Assessing the Health and Social Care Needs of Lesbians, Gay Men and Bisexuals

The legislative framework

Lesbians, gay men, bisexual and transgender (LGBT) people have been among the most socially excluded of minority populations. Arguably, they have faced more legal penalties than any other disadvantaged group. The early twenty-first century, however, has seen a culture shift in the legislative landscape with the removal of almost all of the discriminatory legislation affecting their lives (see Appendix A). LGBT people will be no longer criminalised for behaviour considered 'normal' among heterosexuals and they can begin to participate in public life in ways which were previously debarred to them. The provisions of the Adoption Act 2002 mean that same-sex couples are no longer denied the opportunity to adopt jointly, but are subject to the same criteria as heterosexual couples. The Gender Recognition Act 2003 allows transgendered people to have their birth certificates altered to show their current gender status. Domestic abuse within same-sex relationships has been recognised for the first time in law by the Domestic Violence, Crime and Victims Act 2004. These changes will have a considerable impact upon the civil rights of LGBT people. But the removal of legal sanction is in itself insufficient to achieve lasting benefit in LGBT people's lives; they experience significant inequalities in health and social care and they often face unsympathetic treatment from service providers. What is needed are supportive policy initiatives and practice guidelines.

Developing a health and social policy agenda for LGBT people

Since its election in 1997, New Labour has sought to build a socially inclusive society through a range of policy initiatives; the link between the social, political, cultural and economic disadvantage in people's life circumstances and health and social care outcomes has been acknowledged. In its flagship policies, the government has pledged its commitment to sustaining an ethos of fairness and equity and to the achievement of good health and social care for everyone (Fish, 2005). Furthermore, it is committed to providing information and practical support to improve emotional well-being and access to services.

By contrast, policy-makers have been slow to develop the range of initiatives needed to tackle the social exclusion of LGBT communities. This is partly because lesbian, gay, bisexual and transgender people remain invisible within service provision (see Chapter 6). But it is also because access to relevant data, which is key to the identification of LGBT health and social care needs, is lacking. The scale of this task cannot be underestimated: there are few statistics about sexual identity which could be used to inform policy development. Although data are routinely collected for 'race', gender and disability, population studies such as the General Household Survey, do not record sexual identity and policy-makers do not have the most basic information, such as the size of the LGBT population in the UK. Large-scale studies, particularly favoured by policy-makers, have not been undertaken due to a lack of funding and due to difficulties in conducting research among hidden populations (see Chapter 4). Even government-sponsored initiatives, such as the Department of Health External Reference Group on Sexual Orientation, have foundered because of these barriers. Indeed, in areas where policy initiatives might be expected, the government has failed to recognise LGBT people as service users. The Tackling Health Inequalities initiative made only cursory mention of lesbians and gay men, despite evidence of need, for example, in lesbians' uptake of cervical screening. This is in contrast to policy formulation in the US, where lesbians and gay men are included among groups targeted for reducing inequalities in health outcomes in the US government's public health strategy Healthy People 2010. A significant gap in the policy formulating agenda is research into the needs of transgender people. Despite considerable lobbying by the Gay and Lesbian Medical Association and the production of an extensive dossier (Dean et al., 2000), transgender people were omitted from the US health strategy document. Although Stonewall in Scotland have extended their remit to include transgender people, there is a dearth of empirical research into their health and social care needs. Often when transgender people are included in the project title, it is only a token gesture. For this reason, specific consideration of transgender people's needs is undertaken in Chapter 3.

Notwithstanding these limitations, there is a small but growing body of research conducted among local communities in the UK. These studies provide the framework for the assessment of the health and social care needs of lesbian, gay and bisexual people. This review aims to consider how LGB needs may differ from those of heterosexuals and to consider issues which may limit access to services.

Access to health and social care

A major barrier to equitable health and social care is the lack of information about the specific needs of LGB people. Health and social care provision is based on the concepts and assumptions of heterosexuality. Lesbians, gay men and bisexuals are presumed to be heterosexual; they are assumed to have the same needs as heterosexual people; or they are believed to be inferior heterosexuals. Such values and attitudes influence LGB decision-making when they access to health and social care. Questions that many LGB ask themselves before meeting service providers include: How relevant is knowledge about my sexual identity? Am I likely to feel more, or less, uncomfortable if my sexual identity is known? How easy is it to pass as heterosexual? Do I need advice that is tailored to meet my needs as an LGB person? How accepting is the service provider likely to be? If the service provider exhibits heterosexist behaviour, are they also able to deny me (or make access difficult to) the care I need? Some LGB people will disclose their sexual identity to service providers and receive a positive or neutral reception; some will disclose and receive a heterosexist reaction; others will avoid disclosure (see Chapters 6 and 7).

A recent survey found that only 1 per cent of health professionals were 'out' to their superiors (BMA, 2005); it is not then, surprising, that many patients do not disclose. Although prejudiced attitudes are no longer widespread, the first editorial on lesbian health in the *BMJ* prompted a Bournemouth GP to use biblical verses to condemn lesbianism. While the General Medical Council code of practice does not allow doctors to let their views about a patient's sexual identity prejudice the treatment they give, it does allow doctors to air their views publicly. Doctors' views, however, may influence their professional relationships. One consultant refused to have a nurse on his team because he thought the nurse was gay; and lesbian and gay doctors fear that their career would be jeopardised if their sexual identity became known (Saunders et al., 2000). The undergraduate medical curriculum provides minimal training about LGBT issues. Most medical textbooks make little mention of lesbians, gay men and bisexuals except in relation to HIV, psychiatry and genito-urinary medicine. Such a focus reinforces heterosexist assumptions.

The code of ethics for social workers is more explicit in its commitment to anti-oppressive practice and to challenging sexual identity discrimination. Yet this commitment does not appear to translate into practice. Bayliss (2000) notes that assessments sometimes fail to meet LGB service users' needs because of heterosexist assumptions. Moreover, despite the profession's value base, social workers have not regarded the work as central to their practice: there has been no routine consideration of sexual identity on team agendas or in supervision and, despite being required to provide examples of anti-discriminatory practice in their training, no social work students gave examples of anti-heterosexist practice (Logan et al., 1996). Surprisingly, more research has been undertaken in relation to LGB health rather than social needs. Furthermore, the Royal College of Nurses and the Royal College of Midwives have been pro-active in developing practice guidelines about the health care of LGB people. *Not 'just' a friend* includes information about next of kin issues; power of attorney; registered partners; conflict with other relatives; mental health services; and learning disability. The rest of the chapter seeks to address this gap by including consideration of the social and health care needs of lesbians, gay and bisexual people. It identifies key policy areas for LGB people including community safety; heterosexism and homophobic bullying in schools; domestic abuse; eating disorders; mental health and suicide; substance misuse; sexual health; housing; and parenting. Knowledge about these issues is crucial for the design and delivery of appropriate services.

Community safety

Lesbians, gay men and bisexuals are increasingly visible in British life. Pride events are an important feature of the social calendar and take place throughout the UK; reports about gay issues are now commonplace in the mainstream media; and bars and clubs are no longer hidden away in the alleyways and back-streets of major cities. It would seem that the social climate of the early 1990s is in the distant past, when serial killer Colin Ireland was able to murder gay men with impunity, because police failed to recognise the killings as hate crimes. Although with the introduction of the Crime and Disorder Act 1998 there are now guidelines to identify hate crimes (ACPO, 2000), it would seem that homophobic attacks are on the rise and gay men continue to be murdered in London and elsewhere. High visibility has made lesbians and gay men targets for attack. Contrary to assumptions that places such as Manchester's gay village afford protection and a safe haven for LGB people, Pritchard et al. (2002)

found that the area surrounding Canal Street has one of the city's highest levels of reported assault.

Victim surveys

Prior to the introduction of the legislation, there had been no systematic recording of hate crimes by the police. In order to provide evidence of need, a number of victim surveys were undertaken to document the extent and nature of homophobic incidents. Two large-scale UK national surveys of hate crime (i.e. Mason and Palmer, 1996, N = 4000; Wake et al., 1999, N = 2656) found high prevalence rates of homophobic incidents. Research in Scotland and Wales found slightly higher levels of physical violence and bullying than found in surveys of the UK as a whole (Morrison and Mackay, 2000; Robinson and Williams, 2003). In addition to what is known about nationally, there have been a number of studies of needs assessments (e.g. Brighton, Leicester, Nottingham) which have included questions relating to community safety in local communities.

The prevalence and nature of homophobic incidents

Wake et al. (1999) found little difference in the prevalence of homophobic incidents between gay men and lesbians: 67 per cent of men and 64 per cent of women reported being a victim. The most common incidents were verbal abuse, threats and intimidation and physical assault, but they also included sexual assault and rape, arson and blackmail. There were differences in the kinds of incidents experienced: women were more likely to have experienced verbal abuse; men were more likely to have experienced physical assault. By contrast, younger lesbian and bisexual women were targeted more frequently overall than young gay and bisexual men (Galop, 1998).

There seem to be some differences in the nature of hate crimes throughout the UK. In Scotland, a study of 300 gay men found that 60 per cent of homophobic incidents involved a stranger as a perpetrator. These attacks were not only committed against gay men using 'cruising grounds'. Most occurred when the victim was near or leaving a gay venue, with many incidents occurring in the evening or early morning; moreover, one in four victims felt the perpetrator had identified them as gay because of the way they looked (Morrison and Mackay, 2000). Figures released by the Metropolitan Police suggest that a large proportion of homophobic incidents in London occur in the afternoon and evening. Often, perpetrators were known to the victim as people living in the same neighbourhood.

Avoiding violence

Hate crimes against lesbians, gay men and bisexual people are acknowledged to have a serious effect on the quality of life of their victims.
Like 'race' and disability hate crimes, lesbians, gay men and bisexuals
are targeted because of their identities. The threat of violence extends
beyond the immediate victims; most lesbians, gay and bisexual people
took steps to avoid violence by changing their behaviour in public
spaces (e.g. holding hands or showing affection) and a substantial proportion tried to avoid looking obviously gay (Mason and Palmer, 1996).
In some areas of the UK, LGB people avoid going out at night out of fear
of violence. These solutions to the threat of violence may undermine
the quality of life of LGB people and limit their ability to participate in
public life.

Reasons for reporting and not reporting

A persistent problem is the under-reporting of hate crime to the police;
two studies have found that 82 per cent of all incidents are not reported
(Wake et al., 1999). The most common reasons for not reporting hate
crimes were: perceptions that the incident was not serious enough;
beliefs that the police would fail to take action; and an anticipated heterosexist reaction from the police. People commonly reported hate crime
because of previous experience of a positive police response and the
desire to make the police aware of hate crime in the hope that something might be done. Overall, men were more likely than women to
report incidents to the police; of all the types of hate crime, damage to
property was most likely to be reported. In order to establish whether
there was a potential for over-reporting of hate crime, Morrison and
Mackay (2000) compared the crime rates of so-called 'sexual preference
neutral crime' (e.g. theft from a vehicle and housebreaking) and found
similar or lower rates to those in the Scottish Crime Survey for all males
in the same age cohort.

The Crown Prosecution Service released its first full set of statistics for
hate crimes committed against LGBT communities in July 2005. They
show that in the previous year, the CPS prosecuted 317 cases nationally
with a homophobic element and while the conviction rate appears to be
relatively high – 71 per cent – there is a gap between outcomes for hate
crimes and non-hate crimes. Furthermore, a quarter of cases were dropped
because the victim unexpectedly failed to attend court. These figures
appear to be small when compared to the number of hate crimes reported
to the Metropolitan Police.

Policy developments

The large-scale victim surveys – one undertaken by Stonewall and the other supported by the National Advisory Group for Policing Lesbian & Gay Communities – in addition to the *Admiral Duncan* bombing, were influential in bringing about change in policy in relation to community safety. Hate crime guidelines, introduced by the Association of Chief Police Officers in 2000, the public policy statement launched by the CPS in 2002, and a practice briefing for community safety partnerships – each should contribute to improving police response to homophobic crime, facilitating prosecution of perpetrators and supporting community partnerships to reduce crime levels. In many areas of the UK, hate crimes are the focus of special policing by dedicated community safety units; they have introduced special reporting measures and liaise with local LGB communities.

Heterosexism and homophobic bullying in schools

'Something to tell you': two decades on

Heterosexism is commonplace in schools: lesbian and gay experience is marginalised in school curricula and homophobic bullying is rife among pupils. One of the first studies conducted in the UK among young LGB people investigated 416 teenagers' experiences of schools. *Something to Tell You* explored young people's perceptions of the nature and extent of discussion about homosexuality in school curricula and whether they found the discussion helpful. Nearly two decades later, Ellis and High (2001) replicated the study to identify changes in LGB experiences of education and to consider the effect of section 28 in schools. Despite the repeal of section 28 and more liberal social attitudes, the later study found an increased number of reports of verbal abuse, isolation, teasing, physical assault, being ostracised and being subject to pressure to conform in 2001 in comparison to the 1984 study. Homosexuality was much more talked about in 2001 and while there was an increase in the number who found this helpful, almost 60 per cent said it was not talked about in a helpful way. Research has suggested that the main effects of section 28 were to silence teachers who are supportive of LGB rights; to limit the available teaching resources; and to create an environment where many teachers believe they would be in breach of their employment contract if they discussed homosexuality in the classroom. However, many teachers believed that a morally neutral approach to homosexuality was required of them in order to provide an unbiased education. By contrast, Ellis and High (2001) contend that the approach where teachers do not make their values transparent is flawed.

The ubiquity of 'gay' as a term of abuse

The word gay is the most frequent term of abuse in school playgrounds. A number of studies have investigated the nature and extent of hetero-sexist verbal abuse in schools: in one study, participants reported hearing words like poofter, gay and faggot over 50 times daily. Most work has been conducted on male homosexual pejoratives and the word gay is used as a generic term of abuse in both primary and secondary school environments. While these pejoratives lack sexual meaning in primary school usage, by the time children attend secondary school at the age of 12, the terms have acquired sexual connotations which signify a lack of masculinity. Homophobic abuse is targeted at those boys who are academic, who do not integrate in peer culture or those who conform to adult expectations at the expense of peer group loyalty. Homophobia targets anything that signifies a lack of allegiance to the collective expectation of male peers (Plummer, 2001). The foundations for the negative attributions of homosexuality are laid in childhood and they provide the context for the subsequent sexual identity formation of all men. The severity, frequency, duration and relative power of homophobic abuse exceeds most other forms of verbal abuse and boys rated homophobic pejoratives more seriously than girls.

The consequences of homophobic bullying for young LGB people

Possible outcomes for young LGB include depression and attempted suicide, difficulty in forming relationships, running away from home, unauthorised absences from school and educational under-achievement. Young LGB people may be disproportionately vulnerable (in relation to adults) to abuse and harassment: 78 per cent of those under the age of 18 had experienced verbal abuse and 23 per cent had been attacked by other pupils (Mason and Palmer, 1996). Young LGB people are more likely to experience verbal and physical abuse at school and in the street than in any other location (Galop, 1998). Their experiences of bullying in school were long-term, systematic, and were perpetrated by groups of peers rather than by individuals (Rivers, 2001). Many young people did not report incidents of bullying to teachers nor to someone at home; as adults, some of those bullied reported nightmares or flashbacks related to the bullying (Rivers, 2004).

The introduction of policy to combat homophobic bullying

Recent research has contributed to a climate in which homophobia in schools is acknowledged as a problem that needs to be dealt with (Rivers, 2001). There have been recent policy developments to tackle homophobic bullying in schools: *Stand Up For Us* and *Bullying: Don't Suffer in Silence* offer practical guidance for developing school policies and procedures for dealing with homophobic bullying, checklists to help identify homophobic language and examples of incident logs to record homophobia in schools. There are also suggestions for the ways in which young people may be supported in the coming out process.

Domestic abuse in same-sex relationships

What is domestic abuse and why has it been overlooked in LGB relationships?

Domestic abuse has historically been considered a family issue: overwhelmingly the perpetrators have been heterosexual men and the 'victims' heterosexual women. Typically abuse is endured over a long period – on average 30 incidences – before women report it. It can consist of physical violence, sexual assault and psychological or emotional abuse; and, in extreme cases, it can result in death (Burke and Follingstad, 1999). As a consequence of three decades of feminist campaigning, there is a nationwide network of refuges for (heterosexual) women fleeing their violent partners and a range of support services to enable them to live independently.

Domestic abuse in same-sex relationships is possibly one of the most under-investigated areas in LGB research. It has only recently been recognised in legislation with the introduction of the Domestic Violence, Crime and Victims Act in November 2004. This neglect is partly ideological: beliefs perpetuated by the 1988 Local Government Act that LGB relationships are 'pretend' families have meant that their needs have been ignored by policy-makers. It can also be attributed to an absence of data: the British Crime Survey does not explicitly collect data about the sex of the victim's partners (Gadd et al., 2002). Lesbians and gay men face such particular obstacles in dealing with abuse in their intimate relationships that some have coined the term 'double closet' to describe it. There are a number of reasons which explain the neglect of intimate partner abuse in LGB relationships. Among activists, attention has focused upon violence outside the home: changing the way the police respond to homophobic hate crime and encouraging LGB 'victims' to report it.

There is also the belief that same-sex relationships are inherently more egalitarian and consequently that violence is much less likely to occur within them. Furthermore, many lesbian feminists, in particular, have not wished to draw attention to domestic abuse because of fears that it would further pathologise lesbian relationships. Such fears have some legitimacy; heterosexual women were deemed responsible for abuse and the perpetrator was often exonerated (e.g. she must have provoked him). By contrast, among lesbian couples, it is the relationship itself which is blamed; for example, some suggest that butch-femme relationships cause abuse (i.e. those most similar to heterosexuality); others infer that abuse is likely to be part of a relationship when lesbian partners share all recreational and social activities (i.e. those most different to heterosexuality) (Burke and Follingstad, 1999). Some argue that merger, a condition that gives rise to abuse, is more likely to feature in lesbian relationships. A report on homicide in the UK suggests that gay men are at increased risk of being killed by a current or former partner in comparison to heterosexual women. Twenty-one per cent of men killed by partners were killed by men – these figures far exceed their proportions in the UK population. In terms of the prevalence of domestic abuse, figures are available only for Scotland. The assailant was male in 6 per cent of cases of domestic abuse against men reported to the Scottish police in 1999 and 2000.

Similarities and differences with heterosexual domestic abuse

A key question is whether abuse in same-sex intimate relationships is a unique, or similar, phenomenon to that in opposite-sex relationships. Those issues which appear to be similar are: abuse is said to occur at the same rate as in heterosexual relationships, and there are similarities in the kinds of abuse perpetrated and in some of the personality traits of abusers (e.g. dependency and need for control). But there are also important differences which may prolong and exacerbate experiences of abuse. These include: the threat of outing to family members, employers, landlords and others; male perpetrators persuading their same-sex partner that their behaviour is an expression of masculinity not domestic abuse; undermining sexual identity (not a 'real' lesbian/gay man); internalised heterosexism such as controlling levels of outness; and placing blame for sexual identity (Gadd et al., 2002; Pringle, 2003). Heterosexism in the workplace and from neighbours may also put relationships under stress.

What causes domestic abuse in same-sex relationships?

In heterosexual relationships, domestic abuse is frequently associated with financial issues and it may be that income differentials occur more frequently in heterosexual relationships. In their review of nineteen studies, Burke and Follingstad (1999) found that abuse in same-sex relationships was triggered by the unequal division of household labour; social class differences; decision-making (the batterer was more likely to be the one to make the main decisions); attitudes towards spending money; living in large cities; lower partner education; differences in health status; and use of alcohol (McClennen et al., 2002). The quality of a relationship is associated with the low frequency of abusive behaviours. For gay men, although not lesbians, relationship rituals and maintaining sexual agreements were significantly correlated with quality (Burke and Follingstad, 1999).

Reporting same-sex domestic abuse and access to services

LGB may be reluctant to report domestic abuse because they expect to receive a heterosexist response. Studies have found low levels of reported abuse. There was some limited evidence in Scotland to suggest that the police had been referring assailants in same-sex couples to the Procurator Fiscal less frequently than assailants in opposite-sex couple relationships. Those men who abused male partners or ex-partners were more likely to have had no further action taken against them by the police than those men who abused female partners or ex-partners (Gadd et al., 2002). The lack of service provision for LGB may isolate victims from potential sources of support; for example, there are only 18 refuge places for gay men in the whole of the UK. The new legislation allows same-sex couples to obtain restraining orders for the first time and is aimed at ensuring that cohabiting same-sex couples have the same protection as heterosexual couples. Broken Rainbow is one of the few services dedicated to LGB 'victims' of same-sex domestic abuse and they make a number of recommendations to improve recording systems, training for professionals, funding and resources for the LGBT community and a call for government to provide appropriate refuge provision for LGBT people (http://www.lgbt-dv.org/html/rainbow.htm, accessed 20 April 2005).

Eating disorders among gay men

Similarities and differences with heterosexual women

For the past two decades research has suggested that gay men are at greater risk for eating disorders when compared to both heterosexual men and lesbians. In comparison to heterosexual men, gay men are more likely to engage in recurrent binge-eating and purging and they share similar levels of body dissatisfaction to heterosexual women (French et al., 1996). Some researchers, believing that poor body image is linked to femininity, have used research instruments primarily designed for women. While there do appear to be some similarities to heterosexual women in terms of age of onset, dissatisfaction with current body shape and restrictive dieting methods, in heterosexual women, weight concerns predominate and femininity was not associated with eating pathology in men (Russell and Keel, 2002).

The ideal gay male body shape, by contrast, involves being both thin and muscular. These twin ideals suggest that eating disorders in gay men may differ from those exhibited by heterosexual women and may explain why previous research findings have been contradictory. While gay men are more dissatisfied with their bodies than are heterosexual men, they are no more likely to be heavier than their ideal weight. Rather than being solely concerned with body weight, gay men's body dissatisfaction is related to both the composition and appearance of their bodies. Their self-esteem was lower if they believed that appearance, weight and muscularity were important to others and they believed that their partners preferred a thinner figure. Gay men also believed that increased muscularity would offer protection from physical attack (Kaminski et al., 2005). In the light of evidence of homophobia-fuelled hate crimes this latter belief may well have some legitimacy. However, the twin ideals of thinness and muscularity may pose particular difficulties because the physiological process of building muscle invariably involves accumulating a small amount of fat and the consumption of sufficient calories to permit muscle growth. Gay men may restrain their eating habits in potentially unhealthy ways.

Lesbians and weight issues

While homosexuality in men is itself considered a risk factor for eating disorders (Russell and Keel, 2002), in women, it has been believed to be a protective factor and lesbians are generally thought to have a higher body mass index (BMI) than heterosexual women. Previous studies have found that lesbians weighed more than heterosexual women (Cochran et al., 2001); a comparison study suggested that lesbians weighed more than their heterosexual sisters, had a bigger waist circumference and waist to hip ratio (Roberts et al., 2003). Elsewhere, lesbians reported significantly lower drive for thinness and use of exercise to control weight compared to heterosexual women, but they did not differ from heterosexual women in relation to bulimia, body dissatisfaction or weight concern. In a study of younger lesbian and gay men, lesbians were significantly more likely to report problematic eating; however, they were also more likely than young gay men to believe they had a healthy diet (Coia et al., 2002).

Lack of knowledge about eating disorders and gay men

Despite there being more than two decades of research in this area, it is not widely known that gay men are at risk of eating disorders. There is a need to raise awareness of the risks among community mental health teams and other mental health professionals. The identification of risk factors in young lesbians and gay men may inform early intervention and prevention programmes. In the light of differences in body dissatisfaction between gay men and heterosexual women, alternative approaches to psychological treatment are needed.

Mental health

Psychological distress

Gay men and lesbians reported more psychological distress than heterosexual men and women, despite similar levels of social support and quality of physical health (e.g. King et al., 2003). They were at greatest risk for scoring in the higher range on a structured assessment for common mental health disorders: gay and bisexual men showed higher prevalence of depression, panic attacks and psychological distress than heterosexual men (Cochran et al., 2003). Among gay men, there is a small increased risk of recurrent depression with symptom onset occurring during early adolescence (Coia et al., 2002). In comparison to heterosexual women, lesbian and bisexual women had higher rates of generalised anxiety disorder (Cochran et al., 2003). Among women with depression, lesbians were more likely than heterosexuals to be using prescription medication. While bisexual women had significantly poorer mental health than did lesbians and heterosexual women (Rothblum and Factor, 2001), bisexual men reported more psychological distress than any other group. In accounting for these higher levels of psychological distress, some researchers suggest that poorer mental health may be linked to the increased likelihood of both lifetime and day-to-day experiences of discrimination among lesbians, gay men and bisexuals.

Self-harm

Lesbians were slightly more likely than other groups to have considered self-harm. Among those who had ever considered self-harm, bisexual women were the most likely to have done so (King et al., 2003). Lesbians and gay men were more likely than bisexual men and women to cite their sexual identity as a reason for harming themselves. Coia et al. (2002) suggest that low self-esteem was positively correlated with self-harm in young people. In accounting for these higher rates of self-harm, King et al. (2003) propose that self-harm is less to do with confusion about sexual identity, but rather how to express it openly in society.

Suicide

In the general population, young women more frequently attempt suicide than do young men; however, young men are much more likely to complete suicide. By comparison, young gay and bisexual men may be seven times more likely to attempt suicide than young heterosexual men and Remafedi et al. (1998) suggest that these deaths may explain the increasing rates of suicide among adolescents. Although it is not known whether suicides are more likely to be completed by young gay and bisexual men, multiple attempters are more likely to 'succeed' and reports from psychiatrists suggest that the methods of suicide used by young gay and lesbian adolescents are more severe and lethal than those of young heterosexuals (Remafedi et al., 1998). A study of adult male twins found that on three measures of suicidality, gay and bisexual men scored higher than did their heterosexual twin (Herrell et al., 1999).

Predictors of suicide risk among gay and bisexual men, in comparison with those who have never attempted suicide, include a history of substance misuse, of having been bullied at school, of having lost friends when coming out and of having been sexually assaulted. Some dissatisfaction was reported about the levels of support available. Research conducted for the UK charity Childline suggests a link between suicide risk and homophobic bullying. Black lesbians and gay men were the least likely to report considering suicide (King et al., 2003).

Use of mental health services

Gay men and lesbians are greater users of mental health services in primary and secondary care than heterosexual men and women (King et al., 2003) and gay men are more likely than their heterosexual counterparts to have sought advice from their GP for emotional difficulties. Despite this relatively greater usage of mental health services, lesbians, gay men and bisexuals reported mixed experiences of services: one-third of gay men, one-quarter of bisexual men and 40 per cent of lesbians recounted negative or mixed reactions from mental health professionals when being open about their sexuality (King et al., 2003). In addition, 20 per cent of gay men and lesbians and one-third of bisexual men recounted that a mental health professional made a causal link between their sexuality and their mental health problem. Some have suggested that mental health professionals may be insensitive or hostile to their needs and that service users received discriminatory treatment (Welch et al., 2000).

Disclosure of one's sexual identity (being out) was associated with receiving mental health services among lesbians; qualitative studies have attributed this increased usage to the stress caused by social oppression and lesbians' desire for personal growth.

In one study, over three-quarters of health professionals involved in the assessment and management of adolescents who self-harm were unaware that homosexual young men are at greater risk of deliberate self-harm and one-third of staff were unaware that adolescents who self-harm are at increased risk of suicide (Crawford et al., 2003).

Levels of outness

Disclosure of one's identity to others is usually associated with better mental health, decreased psychological distress and lower suicidality (Morris et al., 2001). Being out is linked with less anxiety, possibly because of the lesser likelihood of involuntary disclosure, greater self-esteem and levels of social support. Rothblum and Factor (2001) contend that the poorer mental health of bisexual women may be related to their decreased likelihood of being out: negative attitudes about bisexuality persist in both mainstream and lesbian communities. While black women were more likely to have self-identified as lesbian or bisexual for longer periods of time than other groups of women, they were less likely to have disclosed their identity to others (Morris et al., 2001).

Substance misuse

Perceptions of alcohol use

There is some controversy regarding the higher rates of alcohol consumption and other substance misuse among lesbians, gay men and bisexuals. Prior to the 1980s, researchers believed that there was a causal connection between homosexuality and alcoholism. Some suggested that lesbians drank to inhibit their abnormal sex drives, despite findings that there are no differences in the amount of alcohol used before or during sexual encounters between lesbians and heterosexual women. Much of the early work was drawn exclusively from bar populations and while these were relatively accessible to researchers, drinking levels were inevitably high. Some explanations point to the central role that bars and clubs occupy in lesbian and gay communities due to the history of exclusion from mainstream social settings. Bars may contribute to greater levels of drinking through simple exposure to alcohol or through cultural norms that sanction alcohol or drug use as a component of social interaction in gay and lesbian communities. Other explanations suggest that heterosexism and homophobia may exacerbate the use of alcohol and other substances as a coping mechanism for dealing with discrimination: one study found that lesbians were more likely to use alcohol to mitigate the effects of workplace harassment than gay men or heterosexual women (Nawyn et al., 2000). Another study found that childhood sexual abuse was associated with lifetime alcohol abuse in both lesbians and heterosexual women (Hughes et al., 2001). While social spaces available to lesbians and gay men are no longer wholly concentrated in bars, these spaces are possibly still the most accessible and may be associated with binge drinking among younger bisexual and gay men. Beliefs that lesbians and gay men have increased rates of problem drinking are pervasive. Even in a study which found comparable rates of drinking between lesbians and heterosexual women, the lesbians in the study were still more likely to believe that lesbians use alcohol excessively (Welch et al., 1998).

Alcohol consumption

Studies among lesbian and bisexual women have suggested that they were more likely than heterosexual women to consume alcohol more frequently and in larger quantities and they were much more likely to be classified as heavy drinkers (Gruskin et al., 2001). Patterns of alcohol use may differ among different groups. For example, while black lesbians are more likely to be lifetime abstainers from alcohol, they are also more likely to report current heavy drinking (Ettorre, 2005). Gay men reported higher overall consumption than lesbians in a US study; however, the findings were reversed in a Swedish study (Bergmark, 1999). Additional drinkers among lesbian and gay male communities appear to fall in the moderate, rather than in the heavy, drinking category and they share between them more similar drinking characteristics than are found in the general population. While the findings about levels of drinking have been mixed, the proportion of lesbians and gay men who abstain from alcohol altogether is considerably less than in the general population (Bergmark, 1999). By contrast, some studies have suggested there are no differences in drinking levels between lesbians and heterosexual women and that heavy drinking or drinking-related problems have declined in recent years (Hughes, 2003).

Alcohol problems

Despite a lack of consensus about their representation in the heavy drinking category, studies appear to confirm that gay men and lesbians have high rates of reported alcohol problems. Studies among lesbians have suggested that they were more likely to report they were in recovery from alcoholism (even when low overall rates were found), they had a greater prevalence of alcohol use problems, greater use of alcohol treatment services and to have wondered whether they might be developing a drinking problem than heterosexual women (Cochran et al., 2001; Hughes 2003).

Smoking

In comparison with US women in general, lesbians appeared less likely to report being current smokers, but more likely to indicate a history of smoking (Cochran et al., 2001; Roberts et al., 2003). In a review of twelve studies of smoking prevalence, lesbians, gay men and bisexuals were found to have higher rates of smoking than in national survey data (Ryan et al., 2001). In addition, black lesbians and bisexual women may be more likely to smoke (Sanchez et al., 2005). Researchers have recommended that LGB communities should be included in future in order to understand the apparent high smoking rates. Attempts should be made to target prevention and cessation interventions to them and they should be culturally sensitive (Sanchez et al., 2005).

Drug use

Gay men and lesbians were more likely than heterosexuals to have used recreational drugs (King et al., 2003). Lifetime cannabis use was high and lifetime cocaine use was doubled amongst lesbians and gay men in comparison to the heterosexual population; no gender differences were found in the homosexual sample. Use of certain drugs, e.g. poppers, appears to be a gay male phenomenon, while lesbian, bisexual and gay young homeless people were more likely to have used injected drugs than a comparable population of young heterosexual people (Noell and Ochs, 2001).

Health outcomes

The effect of problem drinking may be to increase risk behaviour and immunological risk for transmission of HIV amongst gay and bisexual men (Nardone et al., 2001). Men who had used cannabis or inhaled nitrates were more likely to have unsafe sex than those who had not (Clutterbuck et al., 2001). Increased alcohol consumption may be linked to breast cancer in lesbians (Love, 1995) and lesbians' perceptions about alcohol consumption are discussed in Chapter 8.

Substance abuse counsellors have negative or ambivalent attitudes towards LGBT clients, in particular towards transgendered people, and lacked knowledge of their needs (Eliason, 2000).

Sexual health

HIV/AIDS

HIV/AIDS is the most extensively investigated topic within LGB studies; a review of Medline (Boehmer, 2002) found that 52 per cent of all articles published were related to the virus (N = 1958 of 3777). Research funding is a major factor. Since 1982, an average of $20 million annually was spent on HIV-focused work in the US, in comparison to $532 000 on LGB research unrelated to HIV (Boehmer, 2002). HIV/AIDS-related research is also one of the most methodologically varied: in the UK, there have been two population-based studies of sexual behaviour (Wellings et al., 1994; Johnson et al., 2001), a number of large-scale non-probability studies (Elford et al., 2000, N = 1004; Hart et al., 2002, N = 2498) and a range of small-scale qualitative studies have investigated the social context of HIV risk-related behaviour and the psycho-social factors associated with HIV testing (Flowers et al., 2003). Despite medical advances, there is no vaccine for HIV and no cure. The development of antiretroviral drugs has increased the period without symptoms of AIDS, improved quality of life and afforded longer survival. The incidence of HIV is increasing among gay men, however, and some argue that new treatments have reduced concern about infection (Dodds et al., 2005). Safer sex and condom use offer the best protection against transmission of the virus. In the early stages of HIV health promotion, the use of condoms was encouraged for all instances of anal intercourse between men. Subsequently, it became clear that men made decisions about not using condoms based on assessments of their own or their partner's HIV status. Current advice recognises that HIV transmission can be reduced if men have unprotected anal intercourse (UAI) only with partners of the same HIV status. There has thus been a shift from condom use at all times to condom use for sero-discordant UAI – where one partner is HIV negative and one is HIV positive. The numbers of men reporting unprotected anal intercourse has increased, thus negating the benefits of increased condom use (Dodds et al., 2005). Twenty-five per cent of gay men reported unprotected anal intercourse in a three-month period (Elford et al., 2000) and approximately one-third reported UAI in the previous year (Dodds et al., 2005; Nardone et al., 2001).

Knowledge of one's current HIV status is then key to making decisions about UAI; HIV testing for non-clinical purposes is needed if men are to know their HIV status. Yet uptake of testing among gay men is not high: community samples suggest that up to 50 per cent of gay men have never been tested (Hart et al., 2002) and more than three-quarters of men who had never been tested believed themselves to be HIV negative. The GP consultation is an important means of health promotion; however, less than one-third of gay men had discussed safer sex with their GP (Elford et al., 2000). Testing behaviour is associated with demographic factors (e.g. education, age, living in London – Hart et al., 2002; Nardone et al., 2001) and beliefs about the uncontrollability of risk.

Health promotion campaigns should thus be targeted to those at greatest risk: gay men who are HIV negative but in relationships with men with HIV, men with a larger number of sexual partners, and men with lower levels of education should be prioritised in HIV prevention programmes (Hickson et al., 2002). Despite HIV being proportionately more prevalent among gay men, over half of the men in a community survey currently had no personal contact with the virus (Hickson et al., 2002). Approximately 7 per cent of gay men had tested HIV positive.

Lesbians and sexual health

Lesbians have been almost entirely overlooked in debates about HIV/AIDS; the UK's first national Strategy for Sexual Health and HIV fails to mention lesbians and no reference is made to women who have sex with women (Henderson et al., 2002). Because sexual health is conceptualised as the absence of sexually transmitted infections (STIs) and unwanted conception, lesbians are often considered to be the healthiest adult subpopulation. Although it is widely accepted that the efficiency of HIV transmission between women is low, it was only through research into HIV among lesbians in the mid-1990s that the heterogeneity of lesbians' sexual behaviour was first understood. Some bisexual women and lesbians had unprotected vaginal and anal sex with gay and bisexual men and 10 per cent of lesbians and bisexual women were injecting drug users (Lemp et al., 1995). In both of these studies, 1.4 per cent of women had tested positive for HIV. Despite their relatively low risk for HIV, lesbians were more likely than heterosexual women to have ever had an HIV test (24 per cent vs 14 per cent) (Koh and Diamant, 2000). Some suggest that lesbians believe themselves to be essentially invulnerable to STIs because risk is seen to be a heterosexual consideration or on the basis of interpersonal trust. The *National Aids Manual* outlines three risky sexual activities in lesbian sex: oral sex, sharing sex toys and fisting; however, the number of women claiming to have become infected by these activities is at most a handful of cases.

Recent research has been undertaken into lesbians' sexual behaviour and risk of STIs. Approximately 85 per cent of study participants reported sexual histories with men. Bacterial vaginosis (BV) is commonly diagnosed among lesbians (Bailey et al., 2004) and a case-controlled study found higher rates among lesbians than heterosexual women (Skinner et al., 1996); however, it has not been established how BV is transmitted sexually between women. Other STIs such as candida species, genital warts, genital herpes and trichomoniasis were diagnosed less frequently (Bailey et al., 2004).

Housing

The housing needs of LGB communities are not well documented. There is little awareness about the ways their housing needs differ and this is reflected in the provision of housing services: from a dearth of appropriate accommodation for older people to the lack of specialist services for young LGB homeless people. Lesbians, gay men and bisexuals appear to have different patterns of housing tenure from the majority population; they are twice as likely to live in rented accommodation as heterosexuals (Sexuality Matters, 2005). Research conducted in Edinburgh suggests that gay men are more likely to rent their home privately than from a housing association. Because of these differences, LGB people have distinct housing needs: they are more likely to experience a range of problems resulting from insecurity in their housing tenure; they may face eviction and discrimination from housing providers. Gay men, in particular, who seek to become homeowners, may be denied a mortgage or life insurance. It is only recently that research has investigated homelessness among young LGB people. O'Connor and Molloy (2001) outline the causes of the housing crisis and consider the needs of homeless LGB together with their use of services. They recommend the development of specialist services and an inclusive homelessness policy. The Housing Bill, currently before Parliament, proposes to equalise the rights of same-sex couples to succeed to a tenancy.

Parenting

Lesbians and gay men were described as having pretended family relationships in the infamous 1988 Local Government Act. By the turn of the twenty-first century, the family was a key site of debate and social science investigation. A number of arguments were used to dissuade same-sex couples from becoming parents or to limit LGB ability to parent – they were often refused fertility treatment or their applications to adopt were turned down on the basis that they were unfit to parent. Following a bitter struggle, the provisions of the 1988 Act were repealed by the 2003 Local Government Act. In an attempt to appease social conservatives, the government added Sex and Relationship Education guidelines enshrining marriage as the preferred family unit. Many researchers have sought to counter the moral censure of Christian fundamentalists and right-wing politicians by conducting studies to demonstrate that children brought up in same-sex households have similar opportunities for healthy development and are unlikely to suffer because their parents are lesbian, gay or bisexual.

Children of same-sex parents will grow up gay

Most studies have not challenged the implicit heterosexism in this assumption: that growing up gay is less desirable than growing up heterosexual. Instead, longitudinal studies have compared children's development in lesbian mother families with those in one and two parent heterosexual families (MacCallum and Golombok, 2004). Children have been compared for psychological adjustment, socio-emotional development and whether lesbian mothers are more likely to have lesbian daughters and gay sons. Findings suggest that children brought up by same-sex parents are no more likely to grow up gay than children brought up by heterosexual parents. Moreover, the assumption that children's psychological and emotional health is impaired by growing up in a same-sex family has also been refuted.

Children of same-sex parents are bullied

While children are bullied in schools for a number of reasons, the children of lesbians, gay men and bisexuals may encounter bullying because of their parent's sexual identity. Most research has focused upon bullying where children themselves are LGB and there has been little attention to the coping strategies and support mechanisms for children whose parents are gay. Some argue that LGB parents are aware of the likelihood that their child may be bullied at school and are well equipped to help them because of their own experiences. But research suggests that this may be dependent upon LGB parents' own attitudes to their sexual identity, the length of time they have identified as LGB and whether they made the decision to have children in a same-sex or opposite-sex relationship: many LGB come out when their children are in late childhood or adolescence. Some parents are fearful of telling their children: children whose mothers were closeted and uncomfortable about their own sexual identity perceived greater stigma in having a lesbian mother. The cause of these potential problems, however, is heterosexism and not LGB parents or their children.

Children of same-sex couples lack appropriate gender role models

Children brought up by two men (or two women) are assumed to lack the appropriate gender role and emotional behaviour associated with the other sex. This is based on assumptions that men display stereotypically masculine behaviour (e.g. being the breadwinner, assertiveness, interest in sport) and women show only feminine behaviour (e.g. nurturing, passivity, interest in fashion). The fear is that boys brought up by lesbians will be effeminate and that girls brought up by gay men will be tomboyish. The potential for challenging fixed gender stereotypes has largely been ignored. Research has been undertaken, within a conceptual framework that supports heterosexuality, to ascertain the effects on children of being raised in an environment without fathers. Children raised in fatherless families were found to experience more interaction with their mother and perceived her as more available and dependable than their peers from father-present homes. Furthermore, boys raised in families without a father showed more feminine, but no less masculine gender role behaviour (MacCallum and Golombok, 2004). Many same-sex parents are acutely aware of this criticism and take steps to ensure that both sexes play an active part in the lives of their children. Most will have families, friends and neighbours who are included in their lives and a number of parenting groups have been established (such as the Stonewall parenting group in London and others in local communities) to support their parenting needs.

Same-sex parenting

Increasing numbers of lesbians are bringing up children without a male in the household and, while a number of gay men have children, smaller numbers raise children without female involvement. Estimates suggest that a third of lesbians have had children and one-fifth of partnered lesbians have children in the home; the majority are under the age of 18. The number of gay men who are parents is said to be approximately 14 per cent. With changing legislation making it easier for same-sex couples to apply to jointly adopt and loosening of restrictions in fertility clinics, more same-sex couples may make the decision to become parents.

Decisions to parent

There are three main ways that lesbians and gay men can choose to become parents:

Donor insemination

Donor insemination is a method of alternative fertilisation which has been used by lesbians over a number of years. Although the 'science' of alternative fertilisation is relatively simple, more difficult issues are: finding a donor who wants the same level of involvement in the child's life as the lesbian couple want them to have; whether to use a fertility clinic (with the benefits of screening weighed against increased medicalisation); accurately predicting the time of ovulation; and emotional factors.

Surrogacy

Surrogacy may be more likely to be used by gay men. A surrogate mother bears a child for another couple, often by using her own eggs which have been fertilised by one of the men in the couple.

Adoption

Adoption is a legal process where an individual, or a couple, accept parental responsibility for someone else's biological child. Adoption is now open to same-sex parents on the same basis as heterosexual couples. Contrary to popular misconceptions, there are still large numbers of children in the UK who are waiting for a suitable family to adopt them. Most children on the adoption register are not babies, for whom parents can be relatively easily found, but children or young people of school age. Boys over the age of eight are less likely to be adopted than other children and they often remain in residential or foster care. Same-sex couples widen the pool of potential adopters. But they are likely to encounter assumptions about the automatic fitness of heterosexual applicants (Hicks, 2000) which may mean that same-sex couples are less likely to be 'matched' with a child for adoption; the legislation has done nothing to address some of the pervasive attitudes that adoption panels might hold or to provide guidance about matching children and families. Same-sex couples may also need specific packages of support to enable them to provide the best care for their adopted children. In a recent *Channel 4* documentary about adoption, a gay male couple's relationship was compared to being 'best friends' and it was suggested that one of the fathers could be known as the child's uncle.

Conclusion

This assessment provides evidence of some the health and social care needs of LGB people and the issues which impact on their access to services. There are some important omissions; the chapter has not considered the experiences of young LGBT people in care; the needs of the homeless; asylum seekers; refugees; transgender people – who are almost wholly absent from policy initiatives; people in poverty or prisoners (the latter have recently been afforded the same treatment as heterosexuals during domestic visits). Studies of these groups would directly contribute to our knowledge about those who are most disadvantaged in LGBT communities. It has revealed that in many areas of public services, service providers were unaware of the specific needs of LGB people. Knowing about their different needs can help to inform better policy development and better service delivery. Some progress has been made in these areas in particular: policy to address homophobic bullying in schools; practice guidelines for health professionals about the health care of LGB people; and community safety strategy. Yet, despite these important steps, there is an absence of mainstreaming of health and social care provision for LGB people (this issue is addressed in Chapter 9). This is an important limitation and means that policy and practice will be piecemeal and reliant upon the attitudes and innovation of individuals and forward-thinking organisations. Finally, in the struggle to eradicate heterosexism, researchers and activists must be aware of the ways in which the arguments used may contribute to its maintenance. Some research, in seeking to counter the discrimination of LGB, employs the concepts and theoretical assumptions of heterosexism. Not only must we provide evidence that children raised in same-sex families are emotionally healthy, but we must also challenge heterosexist assumptions which imply that growing up gay is inferior.

3
Intersecting Identities: Recognising the Heterogeneity of LGBT Communities

One of the most pervasive stereotypes about lesbian, gay, bisexual and transgender people is that they are white, ablebodied and have large disposable incomes. In LGBT communities, to a much greater degree than any comparable movement, the 'institutions of culture-building have been market-mediated: bars, clubs, newspapers and magazines, phonelines, resort and urban commercial districts' (Warner, 1993: xvii). Traditional forms of association such as local communities, the workplace, churches and kinship networks, schools and colleges have been less available for LGBT people. Much of the early research conducted by LGB researchers was constrained by these realities and inevitably reinforced these assumptions; studies typically recruited LGB who were the most visible and accessible within communities (see Chapter 4) and failed to include transgender people. Yet despite a small but growing field of study among LGB communities, virtually nothing is known about the diversity of the LGBT population. In many studies, groups do not form large enough sub-samples on which to conduct separate analyses and researchers appear to presume that all participants have the same needs (Greene, 2003). Such work is urgently needed because a persistent assumption among policymakers and practitioners is that due to its relative economic advantage, the LGBT population can afford to buy its way out of structural disadvantage by paying for private health and social care.

This chapter aims to challenge widespread assumptions that LGBT communities are homogeneous. Few analyses have been conducted of the ways in which heterosexism functions in relation to youth and age; 'race'; disability; bisexuality; transgender; class; and geographic location. It seeks to identify each group's particular needs in relation to the formation of their identities and coming out; relationships and sexuality; and access to health and social care. Where existing research is available, issues such as mental health and violence have been analysed; in addition, concerns specific to the communities in question are addressed.

Young LGB people

Oppression in the lives of young LGB

Young people are possibly the group within LGB communities on whom most research has been undertaken; yet paradoxically they remain one of the most hidden in society. This invisibility has led one researcher to ask the rhetorical question: 'Are they there?' (Cant, 2003). The societal taboo against homosexuality is particularly acute in relation to young people – reflected in repressive legislation such as the age of consent and section 28 – due to beliefs about the need to protect the young and prevent 'the spread of homosexuality'. Young people are said to be both vulnerable and confused; competing beliefs suggest that young people's emerging gay identities will be fixed in adolescence, and conversely, that being gay is just a passing phase. Because of these assumptions, providers have often been reluctant to offer services (e.g. mental health, eating disorders) for young people and resources tend to be targeted to adult LGB, possibly because it has been too controversial to dedicate provision for adolescents.

Identity formation and coming out

In retrospective accounts, many LGB report alienation, feelings of marginality and difference and the pressure to conform to heteronormative assumptions as teenagers. Adolescence is a period when most young people want to fit in with their peers and the prospect of being different is one that is terrifying to many (Flowers and Buston, 2001). Because they often lack role models in their daily lives and there may be no one in their family, friends or immediate community who may share their experiences, many LGB experience isolation and fear rejection from family and friends. Young LGB people are likely to be more regularly exposed to heterosexist abuse than their older counterparts: in school, on the streets and at home when their social circles are relatively circumscribed and overlapping. Many young gay men, in particular, described childhoods in which they enjoyed solitary activities (reading, music, drawing) rather than the sporting and group activities typically associated with adolescent males (Troiden, 1989). Some had difficulty forming friendships because other boys were reluctant to associate with them from fear that they too would be taunted with heterosexist abuse (Flowers and Buston, 2001). Young lesbians and gay men appear not to socialise with their same-sex peers; both young lesbians and gay men recall that their best friends in childhood were opposite-sex peers. Black young LGB may experience conflict in the development of their identities. One study found that Asian young LGB who endorsed traditional Asian culture and beliefs were likely to face barriers developing a positive lesbian or gay identity because of their culture's rejection of homosexuality. Those who identified as LGB had problems dealing with their Asian identity because of racism (Chung and Katayama, 1998). Young transgender people share some similar experiences with young LGBs; they show a preference for friends of the other sex and for the toys and games stereotypically used by the opposite sex. Most research has been in the form of clinical studies, rather than qualitative studies of young transgender people's experiences of their identity formation and they have found that most wish to belong to the other sex (Di Ceglie et al., 2002).

Troiden (1989), in his classic study of LGB identity formation conducted almost two decades ago, contends that while a sense of being different and set apart from same-sex peers is a persistent theme in the childhood experiences of LGB young people, relatively few label this difference as homosexual when they are children. He found that 20 per cent of young LGB consider themselves as sexually different from the age of 12. The age of knowing they are different, however, may be falling among young LGB. Recent research suggests that by the age of 10, one-fifth of young gay men knew they were homosexual (Sexuality Matters, 2005). Moreover, the majority of young gay men may know they are gay by the age of 12 or 13. This self-identification occurs at a later age for young lesbians, typically 15 or 16. However, young lesbians are much more likely to come out to others at an earlier age than young gay men (18 vs 21) (Coia et al., 2002). The average length of time then, between feeling different and telling someone else may be six years. It is the so-called isolation years which are the most crucial for targeting support and information.

Access to health and social care

Many of the issues around access to health and social care mirror those of LGB adults. LGB young people may be at risk of suicide, drug and alcohol abuse, violence and victimisation, sexually transmitted infections and HIV. Particular issues which are salient for LGB young people are confidentiality issues, information about health and signposting to other services. Most young LGB do not discuss their sexual identity with their health care provider. The small number of those who did disclose received mixed reactions ranging from reassurance that they were normal to the disclosure of their sexual identity to their parents without their consent. Few received safer sex advice and neither they, nor their parents, were referred to a support group.

Older LGB people

Oppression in the lives of older LGB people

The UK has growing numbers of older people in proportion to the rest of the population and older people are generally living longer. Pensioner poverty is increasingly a social problem as few people have adequate pensions to fund (what is increasingly becoming) a longer retirement. Because the UK lacks legislation to prevent discrimination on the grounds of age until December 2006, in comparison to other areas of social policy, there have been fewer initiatives aimed at improving the lives of older people in general. Within a context of less attention, the needs of older LGB have been almost entirely ignored. While there is a substantial body of research, the mainstream gerontology literature largely fails to mention lesbians and gay men. In those few cases which provide discussion, the picture is peculiarly negative. Older gay men have been depicted as lonely, isolated, miserable, with poor psychological functioning and as either sexless or sexually predatory (Pugh, 2002). Moreover, older black LGB are almost entirely absent from the literature (Seneviratne, 1995).

Barriers to disclosure among older LGBs

One of the most common assumptions about older people in general is that they are, and should be, asexual. These assumptions mean that there can be barriers to disclosure that are particular to older LGB, where being non-heterosexual is linked to sexualised behaviour. 'Passing' may be more common among older LGB for a number of reasons: heterosexism in social care assessment and referral forms; older LGB may use different language to describe themselves, such as 'people like us'; and older LGB may have experienced the effects of the criminal and social sanctions that have been only relatively recently removed from statute. In Heaphy et al.'s study (2003) 37 per cent of gay men and 23 per cent of lesbians had hidden their sexual identity throughout their life. In a second study, a gay man changed his name to that of his partner in order to 'pass' as his brother (Langley, 2001).

Older LGB people may also be reluctant to disclose their sexual identity to a home care assistant providing intimate care such as washing or dressing, particularly when they may be attended to by a different care assistant on each day of the week. Conversely, older LGB may feel more comfortable accessing practical support in the form of adaptations to their homes (e.g. following a fall) or in the provision of meals where disclosure of their sexual identity may be perceived to be of less importance. Beliefs that older people are a burden to society may have contributed to health and social care practices which focus on the practical needs of older LGB populations rather than their relationship needs. There are few social spaces dedicated to older LGB and the opportunities for building new social networks may be limited. Moreover, because LGB relationships have lacked legal status, their biological families may make life decisions on their behalf at crisis points in their lives (Bayliss, 2000). There has been comparatively little empirical research which documents the aspirations and needs of service users (for exceptions see: Langley, 2001; Heaphy et al., 2003).

Attitudes and approaches to age and sexual identity

Older people are often seen as a homogeneous group, yet they are a highly diverse population. Among lesbians and gay men, there are sometimes quite different experiences and approaches to ageing. Some men, because they lack the traditional signposts of age – such as children and grandchildren – say that being gay allows them to feel young for longer (Heaphy et al., 2003). Because of the predominance of the commercial gay scene with its youth-oriented culture, however, many gay men say they are particularly conscious of the ageing process and feel excluded from the scene because of their age (Langley, 2001). Lesbians are less likely to have relied on commercial venues for their social contacts and may have developed a range of other avenues to maintain their social networks.

Social networks and informal care

Adjustment to the ageing process is affected by the levels of social support that an individual can draw upon. One perspective suggests that older LGB may have more need of health and social care services because, on the whole, they do not have 'wives [sic] and daughters who make up the usual army of informal carers' (Brown, 1998: 121). Studies among LGB populations in general suggest that they may be more likely to live alone. This may be particularly the case for older LGB; Heaphy et al. (2003) point to the high proportion of older LGB in their study – 41 per cent of women and 65 per cent of men – who lived alone. Partners chose not to live together to protect their independence, to conceal the nature of the relationship, or because the relationship was in its early stages (Heaphy et al., 2003). Coupled with this, almost half saw health and social care professionals as providing care in times of chronic illness rather than partners and family. To counter the effects of isolation in older age, some older black lesbians explored collective ways of living in the future in terms of housing and support (Seneviratne, 1995).

A second perspective contends that 'coming out' is itself a life crisis and that older LGB who have come to terms with their identity and the possible loss of family and friends at the time are better able to cope with ageing. Pugh (2002) argues that older lesbians and gay men have vibrant social lives which involve mutual support; those who are closeted, by contrast, have less support. In comparison to heterosexual men, gay men had significantly more close friends (Pugh, 2002). Lesbians may be more likely than heterosexual women to make the transition to living alone because they are more likely to have had equal domestic relationships, have greater role flexibility and may be skilled in a wider range of domestic responsibilities. If they are bereaved, they may be in a stronger position to continue with day to day existence (Brown, 1998).

Financial concerns

Gender has an influence on financial security in old age. Fewer lesbians than gay men feel they are financially secure. As mothers, lesbians had fewer opportunities to accumulate financial security through an adequate pension and savings. Some women believed their lesbianism facilitated greater financial security because they had no expectations that a male would provide for them (Heaphy et al., 2003). Financial concerns may be exacerbated among older black lesbians and gay men because of the greater likelihood of lower lifetime earnings.

Alzheimer's and mental health

There remains a dearth of practice-based evidence relating to older lesbians and gay men who have mental health problems. Roger Newman, who was a driving force in the establishment of the lesbian and gay Alzheimer's Society Carer's Network, recounts the problems he encountered as his partner's mental health deteriorated. Because of assumptions that HIV/AIDS is widespread among gay men, professionals wanted to test his partner for HIV. Each new encounter with a health and social care professional meant that Newman had to disclose his identity. Gay men, whose partners have Alzheimer's, report difficulties in getting recognition from service providers that they are the most appropriate person to make decisions about their partners' affairs even when they have power of attorney.

Access to health and social care

The greatest fear for older lesbians and gay men was the possibility of going into residential care (Langley, 2001). While this fear may be shared by the older heterosexual population, older LGB people are much less likely to have their needs met. There is no residential care provision for older LGB in the UK and research conducted by Polari (a pressure group for older lesbians and gay men) showed no acknowledgement of their needs by residential care providers. Of greater concern were findings that indicated that many staff in residential homes held heterosexist attitudes. Not surprisingly, almost three-quarters of gay men and two-thirds of lesbians saw care homes as an undesirable option (Heaphy et al., 2003). While most preferred mainstream provision which was LGB friendly, rather than specialist provision, there was notable distrust about being respected in such contexts.

These fears may be well founded due to the lack of privacy afforded in such settings and the attitudes of some workers in care homes. Sale (2002) documents a case where a residential home manager described two older lesbians, who were holding hands while walking along a corridor, as 'dirty pervs'. In a further example, Smith (cited in Langley, 2001: 929) described what happened when a couple tried to hide their sexual identities from the private residential home to which they had moved together when one of them became a wheelchair user after having a stroke. Partners for 50 years, the couple had been found together in the disabled partner's single bed by workers who ridiculed and belittled them. The non-disabled partner had been accused of taking sexual advantage of her confused and vulnerable roommate. The couple were subsequently moved to another home where they had support, respect and a double bed. Such bad practice persists despite the introduction of the policy 'Better Care, Higher Standards: a Charter for Long Term Care' which includes a commitment to counter discrimination on the grounds of sexual identity.

Current day-care provision is designed to meet heterosexual norms. Many older lesbians and gay men do not want to use day-care, but to continue activities with people from existing social networks. This is partly because they can continue to be 'out' about their sexual identity (Langley, 2001). In previous decades, older LGB may have been obliged to pass as heterosexual in their interactions with health and social care professionals. Currently, more people are prepared to live their lives as openly LGB people and this raises new dilemmas for policy-makers (Heaphy et al., 2003).

Policy developments in health and social care for older LGB people

Recent developments in policy and practice promise to offer possibilities for increased choice in LGB people's access to services. Direct Payments (the system whereby a service user employs their own carer) give control to older people so that they can have care provided by a carer whom they employ. In theory, this may mean that older LGB could choose a carer with anti-oppressive and 'gay-friendly' values. In practice, however, its success depends upon the availability of such carers; the system is not well regulated, training for staff is not provided, moreover, social services departments have not actively promoted take up of Direct Payments by older people.

A number of recommendations have been made to improve services for older LGB and develop policies. Policy should address home care, day centres and residential and nursing care and establish a commitment to meeting the needs of LGB older people. Specific examples might help to clarify procedures and practice, for example, where same-sex couples share a room (Kitchen, 2003). Moreover, training for staff should be made available in sexual identity issues including respect for privacy and the use of inclusive language. Social workers should be aware of the existence of relevant support groups, such as the Alzheimer Society's Lesbian and Gay Carers' network.

Black LGB people

Most research among LGB people is conducted with white, middle class participants; furthermore, research about the health and social care needs of black communities largely assumes they are heterosexual. Consequently, the specific needs of black LGB are almost completely ignored and the ways in which racism and heterosexism affect the development of their identities and influence their needs are largely unexplored. Most of the existing literature is North American and although some of the findings may not apply in the UK context (e.g. health insurance), many of the overarching themes may indeed be relevant. The title of this section is not intended to homogenise the experiences of African-Caribbean, African, Middle Eastern, South Asian and South East Asian communities, but rather to foreground them. There are many differences between ethnic minority groups because of different cultural traditions, health status and differences in their experiences of racism and colonialism; however, there are also differences within black groups (e.g. in terms of socio-economic status and education).

There is a common assumption that black communities are more homophobic than white communities and, because of it, black LGB are said to experience such overwhelming difficulties in coming out to their families and friends that many avoid disclosure. Many black communities have strong religious and spiritual orientations and this is often used to attribute higher levels of homophobia. While homophobia undeniably exists in (some) black communities and some black Christians and Muslims use religion to argue that homosexuality should be condemned, the most vocal proponents of religious intolerance in the UK – and those with the most power – are white Christians in mainstream and charismatic churches.

Identity development and coming out: conceptual issues

The literature on coming out experiences and identity formation is probably the most extensive within the field of research on LGB, but it is overwhelmingly about the experiences of white LGB. Moreover, the processes of identity formation and the experiences of coming out may rely, both culturally and conceptually, on western constructs. A key developmental milestone in LGB identity formation (most models use a staged structure) is the disclosure of one's sexual identity to others: in such models greater and greater disclosure is related to greater integrity and authenticity (Harry, 1993). Disclosure to others is seen as so fundamental to the experience of being gay that it is described as the 'gay imperative'; conversely, hiding one's sexual identity implies that an individual is not being 'true to oneself' (Keogh et al., 2004a: 39). The stage model of coming out, however, often confounds two aspects of identity development: the personal (acknowledgement to self) and the interpersonal (acknowledgement to others) and it presupposes favourable social conditions for coming out and finding similar others (Parks et al., 2004). The specificity of black LGB experience means their understanding of their identity, the process of coming out, their behaviours towards others and their values are all infused with the interaction between racism and heterosexism. These issues are explored in the following sections.

Racism, heterosexism and the formation of black identities

Role models are critical for the formation of positive identities: before someone can envisage themselves as LGB they need to see that people like themselves are homosexual and be able to perceive similarities between their own desires and behaviours with those of others known to be gay (Troiden, 1989). A number of books with titles such as *Finding the Lesbians, Inventing Ourselves, What a Lesbian Looks Like* and *Women*

Like Us aimed to meet this need, and while some of them included accounts by black lesbians, they were mainly about white lesbians (for an exception see Mason-John, 1995). Furthermore, many LGB historians have been involved in the project of documenting both the events and the people who have shaped our communities (e.g. Faderman, 1992; Weeks, 1979). Historical figures such as Alexander the Great as well as the derivation of the word 'lesbian' from the time of Sappho have established a sense of continuity. The presence of LGB people in film, mass media, political organising and public life has also contributed to increased visibility.

While a number of writers have made similar attempts to reveal LGB presence in black histories – for example, in the lesbian iconography of Hindu and Jain temples, in the celebration of female power in the goddess Afrekete and the Amazons of Dahomey, and in the tradition of woman to woman marriages in Northern Nigeria and parts of East Africa – they have not achieved parallel visibility. Contemporary role models are equally difficult to find; in a workshop exercise to raise awareness of black LGB, university students were able to name only a dozen black LGB from the UK and the US.

Two of the issues which impact upon the development of black LGB identities are described by Clarence Allen:

> Aligning the two sides of one's life, blackness and gayness, is not always easy: 'I don't think I became fulfilled or rested until the two sides of me met'. It is never easy coming out in a society that, at best, accepts homosexuality on a superficial level (if it is kept secret . . .) and, at worst, physically attacks and sometimes kills lesbians and gay men. Having to open ourselves up to extra abuse or 'allow' ourselves to be doubly oppressed is not done without great thought . . . Forging a black identity is not easy especially when one finds oneself ostracised from the black community for being gay, and from the lesbian and gay community for being black. (Cole Wilson and Allen, 1994: 123–4)

First, aligning the two sides of one's life relates to the process of achieving an integrated black LGB identity. Black LGB sometimes feel they are required to make an either/or choice to identify with either their race or their sexual identity in order to fit in with black heterosexual or white LGB communities (Bridges et al., 2003). In the early years of the feminist movement, black women were often asked to decide which was more important – being black or being female; feminism was thus defined as a white women's issue. Similar demands have been made of black LGB;

those who are perceived to affiliate primarily with black heterosexual communities are said to give preference to their 'racial' identity above their sexual identity. Not only is it impossible to distinguish between multiple identities, but when people are obliged to compartmentalise their identities, they often experience alienation.

Second, being ostracised by both communities compounds black LGBs' sense of alienation. Many black LGB report experiences of racism in the LGB community; in one study, 26 per cent reported discomfort in spaces primarily attended by whites. In addition, a majority of black gay men reported being sexually objectified owing to their race or ethnicity (Diaz et al., 2001). On the other hand, because an authentic black identity is seen as heterosexual, homosexuality is perceived by (some) black heterosexuals as, at best, a white phenomenon, at worst a white disease. One of the most salient myths about black men relates to their ascribed sexual prowess. The one thing that white culture both respects and fears about black men is their masculinity (Younge, 2005). The black athlete and the black entertainer – the few roles available to black men – rely for their acceptance upon the heterosexualised masculinity of all black men. The notion of the black gay man erodes this cultural signifier. There is much invested in black heterosexuality; black homosexuality undermines the one desired status that black men occupy. Black gay men are thus doubly oppressed; their sexual identity is denied by black heterosexuals and their masculinity is objectified by white homosexuals. While the phenomenon of married men having gay sex in private is not limited to one community, the term 'Down Low' has evolved to describe this practice among African-American men (Younge, 2005).

In some UK cities, there are now long-standing and thriving black LGB communities, as evidenced by a range of groups which have been set up to meet their political or social needs and they include KISS, Safra Project, as well as organisations such as the Naz Project and the black LGB community centre. Black LGB people who live in larger cities are increasingly able to live in the specificity and uniqueness of black LGB identities.

While for some black LGB there appears to be a degree of dissonance between their racial and sexual identity (Bhugra, 1997), others suggest there were no significant differences in the sexual developmental milestones of sexual identity or sexual behaviour between black and white young people (Rosario et al., 2004). Of particular interest is the finding that black young people had greater increases in positive attitudes towards homosexuality and in certainty about their sexual identity over time than did white young people. Elsewhere, black lesbians have been found to have been younger when they began to question their sexual orientation, proceeded more slowly in deciding they were lesbian, and then disclosed their identity more quickly compared with white counterparts (Parks et al., 2004).

In the stage model, there is said to be a strong association between identifying oneself as gay and coming out to others; recent research has questioned this link. Morris and Rothblum (1999) conducted a study which examined the degree to which women are distributed on five aspects of lesbian sexuality and the coming out process. Surprisingly, none of them was found to be highly correlated with any ethnic group. However, it was among African-American lesbians that the highest degree of correlation was found and this was between identity as lesbian and sexual experiences with women.

Coming out to others

Coming out, or the public acknowledgement of one's LGB identity, is widely considered to indicate psychological health and developmental maturity (Parks et al., 2004). The presentation of the self as homosexual to an audience is important in resolving the inconsistency between one's own perception of oneself (as gay) and that of others (as hetero-sexual). In the first stages of identifying oneself as homosexual, Cass argues that an individual feels 'alienated from all others and has a sense of "not belonging" to society at large' (1979: 221 emphasis in original). If the individual moves to the next stage, they seek out other LGB in order to alleviate these feelings and to find acceptance (Cass, 1979). The benefits of coming out to others – and socialising with them – lie in the opportunities to meet a partner; the provision of role models; practice in feeling more at ease with oneself as an LGB person; a ready-made support group (Cass, 1979); and validation of the self as LGB. Black lesbians, gay men and bisexuals, however, are said to be less likely to disclose to others and tell fewer people, than their white counterparts, when they do so. In one study, young black LGB people were less likely to be involved in gay-related social activities, they reported less comfort with others knowing their sexual identity and had disclosed their identity to fewer people than white young people (Rosario et al., 2004). Such findings are supported in a small number of other studies; but rather than viewing non-disclosure as far from 'ideal' (Keogh et al., 2004a), it may instead be used by black LGB as a pro-active strategy. Below, I consider how coming out may be differently experienced by black LGB.

Harry (1993) suggests that the pattern for disclosure that most (presumed white) people adopt is one where some people know about one's sexual identity and others do not. Most LGB make decisions about coming out based on the degree of overlap or communication between audiences before coming out to any of them, and on whether their given audience (neighbourhoods, work colleagues, friends) is replaceable. Black social networks tend to be more extensive and seamless than white networks so that a degree of overlap between audiences is more likely. Given the smaller size of black communities, as a whole in the west, black social networks may be less replaceable. There are also few cities in the US (and in the UK) with sufficiently large black LGB communities to come out to. In addition, the sense of alienation experienced by young white LGB that Cass (1979) alluded to is likely to be compounded for young black LGB because of racism.

Telling others about one's sexual identity or any public expression may incur prohibition: sexuality and sexual expression is a private matter in some cultures (Chan, 1996). According to Gomez and Smith, it is not the behaviour itself that is sanctioned, but its public articulation: 'Play it, but don't say it. That's the sentiment that encapsulates the general stance of the Black community on sexual identity' (1994: 189). There may also be differences within and between ethnic groups in patterns of disclosure and non-disclosure. In one study, a number of African-American gay men reported that while their families knew they were gay, many had never discussed it (Adams and Kimmel, 1997). Other study participants were more likely to have sexual contact only with other white men so that no one in their community would learn of their sexual orientation (Adams and Kimmel, 1997). In order to limit the number of people to whom they disclose some black LGB compartmentalise their identities. For example, some South Asian gay men made concerted attempts at concealment and were likely to hide their sexual identity from work colleagues by acting straight, talking about girls, asking female friends to ring them at work and using other smoke screens (Bhugra, 1997). In another UK study, Asian people were far less likely than those from other ethnic groups to be open about their sexual identity to anyone but their close friends. For instance only 27 per cent of Asian respondents were open to their mothers about their sexual identity compared to 61 per cent of African-Caribbean respondents (Galop, 2001).

The benchmark used to assess LGB identity formation has often been a white model; these issues suggest that the model may not adequately reflect the specificity of black LGB identities.

The role of black families and the legacy of colonialism

The 'coming out' model is based on western concepts of self. In contemporary western cultural traditions, the greatest obligation and duty is to oneself: coming out is a strategy which affirms the self in the world. In other cultural traditions, the concept of an individual identity may not exist in the same way and the immediate and extended family are at least (if not more) important (Chan, 1996; Chung and Katayama, 1998). Decisions about choosing a partner are not merely based upon meeting individual needs, but about a relationship that will bring benefit for both families. In some cultures, the family forms an economic unit that relies on traditional gender roles for the continuation of the family line. For many black people, the family is a site of resistance against white oppression: it is the primary social unit which functions as a refuge against racism and where strategies for dealing with racism are learnt. Coming out may be less valued by black LGB because it might jeopardise the support they need as members of a racial minority and because they cannot presume acceptance by the wider white LGB community because of racism.

Black lesbians appear to be more likely than white lesbians to maintain strong involvements with their families, to have children, to have continued contact with men and their heterosexual peers and to depend on family members for support. Some argue that because of the strength of family ties, lesbian family members may not be rejected, even though there is an undisputed rejection of a lesbian sexual identity. The legacy of forced sterilisations and abortions, the use of the contraceptive implant Depo Provera and unwanted hysterectomies mean that in many black communities the most important obligations are the continuation of the group's presence in the world. Lesbian, gay and bisexual identities are seen, by many people, as incompatible with parenthood. In the historical context of colonialism and slavery, the decision to adopt an overtly gay identity could be viewed as a repudiation of one's ethnicity (Greene, 2003).

Religion

The church has been an important institution in African-Caribbean communities and a potent source in liberation theology (Greene, 2000). Religion plays a central role in many black communities, forming an important part of social and cultural life. For some, membership of faith communities is connected to the process of migration; it is a means of strengthening bonds made in the country of origin, affirming identities and building social networks. Many black LGB people continue to perform regular rituals and prayers (Bhugra, 1997; Keogh et al., 2004a). While some may have difficulty in relating their religion to their sexual identity, others find ways of reframing their religion within a sexual identity affirming paradigm. There is a small body of work which seeks to reinterpret Islamic sources which seem to censure homosexuality (retrieved 15 July 2005 from http://www.safraproject.org/; Yip, 2005). These researchers point to the development of progressive Muslim scholarship which returns to the Qur'an as the most important text on which to base a Muslim moral framework that incorporates homosexuality.

Intimate relationships

Personal relationships are vital to psychological and physical health and longevity (Peplau et al., 1997). In his study of mainly white same-sex couples, Harry (1993) speculated that, unlike heterosexual couples who tend to be demographically similar, there would be less similarity among gay male partners because of the smaller pool of available people. He found that white lesbians were matched on age and education and marginally on income whereas gay male couples were similar only on age. Subsequent research has shown that African-American lesbians and gay men share a fair degree of demographic similarity with their partners. There were also differences between black lesbians and gay men: black gay men reported an average income of over $5000 more than black lesbians, despite similarities in occupational status (Peplau et al., 1997). Other findings suggested that black gay men were considerably younger than lesbians in their age of first same-sex experience (15 vs. 19 years). In addition, black lesbians reported significantly more education and they lived together for longer periods than black gay men.

Black heterosexual people's experiences of health care

Since publication of the *Black Report* (1979) health inequalities have been a key concern for researchers. Townsend and Davidson (1979) contested the cultural deficit model which attributed ill health to the lifestyles, health behaviours or eating habits of individuals. Instead, they suggested that wider social factors might influence patterns of health inequalities such as housing, poverty and race. Notwithstanding growing awareness of the role of wider determinants in health, black people's increased likelihood of unemployment or insecure employment, poorer housing and lower incomes together with their experiences of racism are often overlooked as contributory factors in their poorer levels of health. Furthermore, black people's access to health care is circumscribed by racist ideologies and research has often privileged interpretations which locate health inequalities in black people's culture or genetics. Studies have found lower satisfaction rates among black service users because of inappropriate service provision, a lack of cultural competence of health service staff, western conceptualisations of health and social care and stereotyping of black service users and their families (McLean et al., 2003). Not surprisingly, the expectation and experience of racist mistreatment discourage early access to services; by the time black service users come to the attention of service providers they may be more likely to be in crisis. While relatively little research attention has been devoted to black heterosexual people's access to health and social care (Chiu and Knight, 1999), even less has been given to the needs of black LGBs. This analysis of the unique health and social care needs of black LGB is drawn from the few studies devoted specifically to them in the US and the UK.

Black LGB relationships with health and social care providers

Health care providers hold a range of prejudiced attitudes towards black service users as less educated and intelligent and more aggressive (Malebranche et al., 2004; McLean et al., 2003). These stereotypes may determine diagnosis, type of treatment and the quality of after care. They may also influence service providers' expectations of black service users as more likely to engage in risk behaviours and less likely to be compliant with medical advice. Providers' assumptions can also be communicated by their behaviours which black lesbians detected in body language, facial expressions and gesture; intonation can also convey cautiousness, discomfort and disapproval (Stevens, 1998). Alongside the pathological assumptions of some health care providers, in many areas of service delivery, service providers adopt a colour-blind approach. The only difference acknowledged by service providers appeared to be skin colour: the needs of black service users were viewed as interchangeable with those of the white population (McLean et al., 2003). By contrast, in other areas of health service delivery, 'culture clash' explanations are employed to account for the high rates of self-harm among young South Asian women. This is despite the similarities between their experiences of childhood sexual abuse, emotional and physical abuse and those of white young women. Such explanations contribute to the possibility that vulnerable service users may be advised to contain their problems within the family; the view is often expressed as: 'they look after their own don't they?'

Black lesbians and gay men may be likely to encounter both racism and heterosexism in their receipt of health care. In one of the few studies to specifically address the needs of black gay men, the researchers explored the ways that racial and sexual discrimination influence access to health care, HIV testing, communication and adherence behaviours

(Malebranche et al., 2004). Black gay men's experiences of discrimination fostered feelings of detachment. Some of them expected discriminatory treatment and consequently they viewed the health encounter as a functional interaction limited to 'fix(ing) whatever ails me' (Malebranche et al., 2004: 100). Others set high expectations not only for non-judgmental care, but also to be accepted and valued as a black gay man. The study made several recommendations for improvements to health care for black gay men which included: increasing the number of ethnic and sexual minority providers; expanding current definitions of cultural competency curricula at academic institutions; targeting future research efforts on black gay men; and improving structural and communication barriers.

Access to health and social care provision

There are few studies which investigate access to public sector services by black LGB. The Safra Project conducted research into the needs of lesbian and bisexual Muslim women and found that there was a lack of relevant and accessible information to meet their needs (retrieved 15 July 2005 from http://www.safraproject.org). Moreover, many Muslim LGBs avoid mental health services because of the derogatory perceptions of Islam held by non-Muslim counsellors. The lack of representation of black groups on health services staff is seen as a reason for the low access to mental health services. They also found a lack of appropriate housing for Muslim LGB, who often lived in unsuitable housing or were homeless: less than 0.3 per cent of London's hostels and accessible housing was dedicated to LGB. By contrast, another study showed that black LGB people were more likely to find targeted LGB housing services useful (84 per cent) than they were for other specialist services (Galop, 2001). The Galop (2001) study also asked respondents about their experiences of policing, crime and harassment and it is possible to make some comparisons with a national study: *Breaking the Chain* (Wake et al., 1999). Black LGB were more likely to experience physical abuse than LGB in the national study (24 per cent vs. 14 per cent); more likely to experience harassment from a stranger (70 per cent vs. 60 per cent); and they were equally likely to have endured verbal abuse (30 per cent vs. 29 per cent). However, the participants in the Galop study were much more likely to have reported their victimisation to the police than were the participants in the national study (74 per cent vs. 18 per cent). In the light of black people's well-documented experiences of the police, this is a surprising finding which warrants further study. It is likely that services do not meet the needs of black LGB people who have been victims of violence.

Black gay men and HIV/AIDS

Research on HIV/AIDS is by far the largest topic within the field of LGB studies as a whole, accounting for 52 per cent of research output (Boehmer, 2002). While reporting of participants' race/ethnicity has doubled from 7.8 per cent to 16 per cent between 1980 and 1999, most of this increase is attributed to STI-focused research (Boehmer, 2002). Studies suggest that African-Caribbean men who have sex with men are disproportionately affected by HIV (Malebranche et al., 2004). Compared to white gay men, African-Caribbean men were 2.06 as likely to be living with diagnosed HIV infection, while Asian men were less likely to be doing so (Hickson et al., 2004). In a study in three US cities, Latino gay men, who reported more instances of social discrimination and poverty, were more likely to participate in difficult sexual relations and engage in sexual risk behaviour (Diaz et al., 2004). Despite this increased risk, African-Americans with HIV/AIDS used fewer outpatient services which may result in worse health outcomes (Malebranche et al., 2004). In terms of the socio-psychological impact of HIV status on the intimate relationships of black LGB, Peplau et al. (1997) found that it was not related to relationship satisfaction.

Mental health

Among the black population as a whole, mental health problems are a serious concern. African-Caribbean people are far more likely (in some studies as much as ten times) to be diagnosed with schizophrenia than their white counterparts. African-Caribbean people also suffer higher rates of involuntary detainment in secure psychiatric settings and greater police involvement in sectioning. Minority ethnic communities are far less likely to be offered counselling and tend to be prescribed higher drug dosages (McLean et al., 2003; Matthews and Hughes, 2001). Pervasive stereotypes portray African-Caribbean people as dangerous, threatening and irrational (McLean et al., 2003). Studies among LGB populations have found that, in comparison to heterosexuals, they report more psychological distress, including anxiety, depression and suicidal behaviour. Increased levels of psychological distress may be linked to LGBs' experiences of discrimination (King et al., 2003). While black LGBs' mental health difficulties are said to be directly related to their experiences of oppression (Diaz et al., 2001), caution should be exercised in assuming that multiple minority statuses are indicators of increased risk (Consolacion et al., 2004). A study among black lesbians found that they had developed active coping strategies, including internal strategies of self-esteem, race and lesbian identification with external mechanisms of social support and access to LGB resources (Bowleg et al., 2004). A study which examined multiple minority statuses and psychological health among adolescents found that white young women reported more suicidal thoughts, higher depression and lower self-esteem compared with male adolescents in their racial/ethnic group. Same-sex-attracted youths did not consistently demonstrate compromised mental health across racial or ethnic groups (Consolcaion et al., 2004).

Disabled LGB people

Disability oppression

Disability stereotypes are difficult to challenge because unlike other prejudiced attitudes, disability labelling is seen as benign. Central to these beliefs are notions that disabled people are dependent on care, are less worthy, are childlike, have limited options and are sick. If disabled people are perceived as sick, the corollary is that they should get better; that is, the role of a disabled person is to become less disabled and less dependent. The cost of being considered childlike is to be treated as lacking the adult characteristics of sexuality and autonomy. By contrast to mainstream conceptions in which care is associated with nurturing, disabled people sometimes experience care as oppressive. The practice of overprotecting disabled people places limits on their self-determination and autonomy. Further, disabled people must often endure persistent questioning about their disability that would not be acceptable in other circumstances. Disability scholars draw distinctions between individualised and medicalised conceptions of health, which are attributed to an impairment of the mind or body, and a social model of disability, which is produced through disabling environments and attitudes (Shakespeare, 1999).

Coming out as disabled and gay

Disability erases other dimensions of social experience: assumptions are that disabled people are white and heterosexual. In one study, disabled lesbians felt they were invisible within the disability movement because of their sexual identity and within the lesbian, gay and bisexual movement as disabled people. Most venues where lesbians meet are inaccessible and there is a body beautiful culture which can exclude disabled lesbians (Ellis, 1995). Black disabled lesbians were not 'out' in black communities and were reluctant to be out within the lesbian and gay movement or disability movement. Lesbian disability activist, Kath Gillespie-Sells (1998), suggests that there are parallels between coming out as disabled and coming out as lesbian; for some, being able to deal with one 'difference' helped in coping with the other (Shakespeare, 1999). For others, one identity assumed salience: people denied the LGB aspect of themselves or were not able to assume a social identity as a disabled person. However, others adopted a composite LGB, disabled identity. There are also important distinctions between the two identities. Unlike gay communities in the UK, there is not a broad-based disability community, but rather a movement in which disabled people come together for campaigning rather than leisure purposes (Shakespeare, 1999). The deaf community is an exception to this; local deaf clubs provide an important cultural and leisure resource.

Many disabled people are not able to come out because they live in residential accommodation or with their parents, on whom they may be dependent for care or services.

The social circumstances of LGB disabled people

Lesbian gay and bisexual disabled people (like other people with disabilities) tend to be of low economic status. As disabled children, some experienced a disrupted education; in addition, special schools were seen to provide a second-class education. Disabled children who were educated in special schools, separate from mainstream education, were removed from their immediate social networks (Shakespeare et al., 1996). The lack of education and vocational qualifications means that disabled people are often unprepared for the workforce. The situation is compounded by discrimination on the part of employers; most disabled people are not in paid work, are living at home, or in caring situations and they rely on state benefits (Gillespie-Sells et al., 1998). Many disabled lesbians were denied the opportunity of a career or economic independence. Those who relied on benefits often lived in poor housing and had poor diets. All of these factors are indicators of poor health. Moreover, work not only provides the financial means to have a social life, but it also provides the opportunity for friendships or potential partners. Society also enforces compulsory celibacy by denying disabled people access to relevant and appropriate sex education. In one study, only 28 per cent of disabled women who had attended special schools had received sex education and those who were born disabled were much less likely than those who became disabled to receive sex education (Gillespie-Sells et al., 1998). Many disabled people internalise these assumptions and believe that sex is not for them.

Relationships and sexuality

The possibility of a satisfying sexual relationship is something that most people take for granted, but for disabled lesbians, gay men and bisexuals there is an expectation of compulsory celibacy. Sex and intimacy are not seen as basic needs for a disabled person, but as luxury desires. Despite recognition of the importance of sex for self-esteem and a self-determined life, disabled people are not only perceived to be asexual, but also frequently compelled to be so. There are a number of preconceptions about disabled people's sexuality: all sex is heterosexual; only independently functioning disabled people can handle sexual relations; disabled people should be grateful for a sexual relationship; disabled women cannot be mothers and if they do, their children are not getting a 'real' mother. Alongside these beliefs are concerns that people with a learning disability may not have the capacity to consent to sex and heterosexist assumptions that gay men with learning disabilities may be abused by non-disabled gay men.

Learning disabled LGB people

There are few studies about the health and social care experiences of LGB disabled people and even less about the particular experiences of lesbian, gay men and bisexual people with learning disabilities. Service providers hold contradictory beliefs about learning disabled people's sexuality; on the one hand they are perceived to be asexual, while on the other, they are held to be hypersexual. Access to, and the language of, health promotion materials is inappropriate for people with learning disabilities; targeted materials are likely to be restricted to heterosexual sex.

   Having a sex life is a problem for many people with learning difficulties. In many settings, carers and staff actively discourage any form of heterosexual sexual activity between service users: the disapprobation is more severe if those relationships are same-sex relationships. Yet despite the pervasive heterosexuality of their living environments, men with learning difficulties may be more likely to find male sexual partners because opportunities may present themselves more readily. The fear of a woman with learning difficulties becoming pregnant often results in stricter rules around contact between opposite sexes, whereas it is common for men to share bedrooms and toilets. But while men with learning disabilities may engage in same-sex sexual behaviour, they do not necessarily come out as gay men. There are a number of reasons why men may not disclose: for some the label 'learning disability' is challenging in itself; others do not know what being gay means. Alternatives to heterosexual role models are not readily available; many LGB staff are cautious about coming out to clients because of fears that allegations may be made against them and sensitive to the possibility that they will be accused of imposing their sexual identity on a client. Gay men with learning disabilities may live with their parents; by contrast, many people first come out in environments outside of their immediate family context. Those who live in residential accommodation may have contact with multiple carers: coming out to several people may be particularly daunting.

General practice staff hold stereotypical attitudes about women with Down's Syndrome as irresponsibly sexually active and in need of control or that women with learning disabilities had no access and no desire for sex. Some learning disabled people have internalised assumptions that sex is not appropriate for them and that homosexuality is dirty and dangerous. Same-sex relationships among gay men with learning difficulties are often raised by staff only after they have been identified as a problem, for example, when a service user has been seen using public toilets or has approached another man in a home. Because there are no policies about sexual identity, social care workers often do not know what advice and support they can offer.

There are, however, some examples of good practice to draw on in developing policy and service delivery. Shirley Leggott, a 37-year-old woman with a learning disability, wrote about her experiences in *The Guardian* of coming out as gay and the support she received from the staff where she lived in Mencap-supported accommodation.

Deaf LGB people

Groups for deaf LGB have existed in the UK for over a decade in Brighton, Newcastle, Leicester, Nottingham, London, Derby and Glasgow, and they offer advice and social support to local communities. Deaf LGB have lobbied the national organisation, the British Deaf Association, to include LGB in their equal opportunities policy. Deaf LGB have organised workshops in HIV and sexual health, counselling and befriending, where deaf LGB people themselves have acted as trainers (Nyman, 1991). Despite their relative politicisation and visibility, however, virtually no research has been conducted into their health and social care needs.

Disability hate crimes

Section 146 of the Criminal Justice Act 2003 makes hate crimes against disabled people and lesbians, gay men and bisexuals an aggravated offence. In cases where an offender shows hostility towards a victim based on their actual or perceived disability, learning difficulty or sexual identity, the courts will be able to impose tougher sentences. Despite these legislative changes, the criminal justice system has yet to develop an effective strategy to monitor and respond to hate crimes against disabled people. There are no mechanisms for identifying and recording hate crimes that are perpetrated on disabled people. Moreover, some police forces mistakenly believe that social care has the lead role, through the *No Secrets* policy, in protecting vulnerable adults from abuse. Hate crime against a disabled person is frequently minimised as 'bullying', 'abuse' or 'kids being mean' (Perry, 2004). These terms exacerbate the under-reporting of disability hate crime and compel the victims to change their behaviour rather than supporting them to take action and report the matter to the police.

Access to health and social care

Disabled people may access health care more frequently than non-disabled people and they may be more likely to be subjected to routinised treatment. Despite their potential greater use of health care services, it is only recently that a study (supported by the Disability Rights Commission) has been designed to investigate access to health care by disabled lesbians, bisexuals and gay men (www.regard.org.uk, retrieved 20 April 2005). A US study found evidence of negative attention on the part of health care workers: withholding pain medications, ignoring call lights, staff being cool and detached, and disabled LGB patients being discussed in hushed tones during shift changes (O'Toole and Bregante, 1993).

Karen Shook reflects upon her need, as a disabled lesbian, for social care and whether the social worker undertaking her assessment and making decisions about her future will consider her needs without making judgements about her life. She says:

> But will the people who arrive be respectful and non-judgmental about the books and magazines that I read, the friends that I have, and the way I choose to spend my time? Will they appreciate that I need assistance to attend the lesbian, gay and bisexual Mardi Gras festival or the meetings of the organisation of disabled lesbians, gay men and bisexuals of which I am chairperson? In the past, I have had some very humiliating experiences, when home helps have seen it as their duty to lecture me on the evils of homosexuality. (Retrieved 20 June 2005 from http://www.communitycare.co.uk)

Direct Payments may, however, give her the freedom to employ people of her choosing who will be able to provide her with appropriate support.

Bisexual men and women

Bisexual oppression

Bisexuality has often been characterised as a transitional phase in coming out as a lesbian or a gay man and as a stepping stone en route to another (more secure) identity, rather than an end in itself. This conceptualisation has been in part created by models of sexual identity which were either dichotomous (lesbian or gay) or scalar. In the first, bisexuality was considered non-existent; in the second, most notably the Kinsey scale, bisexuality was located in the middle of a seven-point scale between heterosexuality and homosexuality. Bisexuality, then, is seen as an unstable form of sexuality where individuals switch back and forth between sexual identities. In popular discourses, bisexuals are seen as serial monogamists who alternate between same- and opposite-sex partners, or worse, as promiscuous, and engaging in sex with both genders at the same time. In common misconceptions, a person has to be a perfect hybrid to be truly bisexual: their bisexuality has to consist of exactly equal parts of heterosexuality and homosexuality. Bisexuality, in such formulations, is a third and intermediate category of sexual identity. In most depictions, however, bisexuality is not an identity at all, but rather sexual behaviour. Bisexuality, to an even greater extent than for homosexuality, is a sexualised category.

Bisexuals, lesbians and gay men share a common oppression structured by heterosexism. But when bisexuals turn to the lesbian and gay movement for support and solidarity, they often meet with a mixed reception. Bisexuals have sometimes been accused of trading on heterosexual privilege, of being part-timers who appropriate the resources of the lesbian and gay movement or of betraying lesbians and gay men – either collectively or individually – by sitting on the fence. Bisexuals are only considered to be oppressed when they express their same-sex sexuality; the rest of the time, they are considered to be indistinguishable from heterosexuals. Bisexuals say that lesbians and gay men have stolen their role models (Laird, 2004); and, because one tends to infer a person's sexual identity from the gender of her or his partner, they are the most invisible of the 'queer alliance'.

Bisexuality has the potential to end sexual categories because it poses a unique challenge to the institution of heterosexuality. It is fluid while heterosexuality and homosexuality are fixed. Monosexuals choose their romantic partners on the basis of their biological sex; for bisexuals however, biological sex is only one of a number of different criteria that might be important in selecting a partner (Esterberg, 2002). Bisexuality in its questioning of the rigid hetero/homo distinction obliges lesbians and gay men to rethink modes of organising politically around a class or an ethnic model of identity. Bisexuality also has potential as an inclusive sexuality: it is an identity that (some) black non-heterosexuals may be more likely to embrace.

Identity formation and coming out as bisexual

Because their sexuality does not fit into the straitjacket of the existing dichotomous model of sexual identity, many bisexuals might initially discredit their same-gender feelings in order to maintain a heterosexual identity or ignore their opposite-gender feelings and identify themselves as lesbian or gay. For some bisexuals, their emotional feelings for men and women differ from their sexual feelings. Moreover, because there are a number of dimensions to sexuality, some have proposed a model that takes account of sexual attraction, sexual behaviour, sexual fantasies, emotional preference, social preference, self-identity and lifestyle (Rust, 1997). On each of these dimensions, an individual may occupy different points ranging from other sex only to same sex only. Multidimensional models are useful for recognising the complexity of sexuality and experiences.

Research into bisexual identity formation suggests that bisexual women experience coming out milestones at older ages than lesbians; however, bisexual and lesbian women experienced similar psychological events in almost identical order. Bisexual women first felt sexually attracted to women at an average age of 18, while lesbians experienced these feelings at the earlier age of 15. The coming out process happened more slowly for bisexual women than for lesbians. This delay needs to be understood in a context in which role models for bisexuals are lacking and the difficulty of coming out in a culture which dichotomises sexual identity and behaviour.

Research on identity formation is useful for two reasons: it contributes to the increasing visibility of bisexuality and its cultural legitimacy and it offers a category for political mobilisation.

Bisexuals and HIV

HIV/AIDS has contributed to the increasing visibility of bisexuality; this has largely been because bisexuals have been considered to be the 'vector' in the spread of HIV to the heterosexual population (Champion et al., 2005). Such beliefs have fuelled research into the sexual behaviours and perceptions of HIV risk, predominantly of bisexual men and, to a lesser extent, women. One study showed that a third of bisexual men engaged in unprotected penetrative sex with male partners, while two-thirds engaged in unprotected vaginal sex with female partners.

Research among bisexuals needs to question taken for granted assumptions about their lives. One study suggested that bisexual women engaged in more high-risk sexual behaviours than heterosexual women, including multiple or concurrent partner relationships with both men and women. Given that the sample included only 23 women, it is difficult to see how the researchers concluded that bisexuals form an extremely high risk population of women (Champion et al., 2005).

Mental health

A large-scale study of mental health and social well-being, conducted on behalf of the mental health charity MIND, included 85 bisexual men and 113 bisexual women (King et al., 2003) and is one of the few studies to disaggregate the health of bisexuals. Bisexual men reported more psychological distress than gay men and they were also more likely to have recently used recreational drugs. Bisexual women were more likely than lesbians to recount mixed or negative reactions from mental health professionals when being open about their sexual identity. Bisexual men and women were less likely to have parents or siblings who were aware of their identity than their lesbian and gay counterparts and less likely to be open to colleagues, GPs and mental health professionals. One-third of bisexual men – more than for any other group – stated that a mental health professional made a causal link between their sexual identity and their mental health problem. Gay men and lesbians were more comfortable with their identities than bisexual men and women. Other studies have found that bisexuals had more current adverse events, greater childhood adversity and a higher frequency of financial problems. Bisexual men and women may be at increased risk for suicide.

Substance use and misuse

In a study which compared the prevalence of substance abuse among bisexual and heterosexual women, bisexuals were more likely to report cigarette smoking, illicit drug use and medically prescribed anti-depressant medication. Although their drinking behaviours were similar, bisexual women were more likely to report problems with alcohol (McCabe et al., 2004).

Access to health and social care

Although bisexual men and women are increasingly included in research on the health and social care needs of non-heterosexuals, most studies fail to address their needs separately. Consequently, their needs are largely undifferentiated from those of lesbians and gay men. The problem is further compounded by the increasing tendency of biomedical research, in particular, to use the term men who have sex with men – or the corresponding term for women – and this has led to some confusion in terminology (see Chapter 9 for further discussion).

Transgender people

Cultural constructions of gender

Western cultural traditions divide the world into a dichotomous sex system – male and female – of which everyone is incontrovertibly a member from birth. Genitals are said to be the defining feature of sex: being male depends upon the possession of a penis and being female is determined by the presence of a vagina. To be accepted as an authentic member of either sex, there must be congruence between sex (hormones, anatomy and chromosomes), gender identity (e.g. self-perception and behaviour as male or female) and gender role (e.g. how others perceive an individual). The genitals are said to be the most significant marker of gender identity; but it is the penis, in particular, which determines how gender should be attributed. The 'natural attitude' is to see someone as female only if you cannot see them as male (Kessler and McKenna, 2000). In most cases, however, we make decisions about a person's sex/gender without having seen their genitals, but rather on the basis of a number of other secondary sex characteristics (e.g. breasts, Adam's apple, voice pitch) or presentation (mannerisms, clothing, activities). Knowing someone's gender determines how we relate to them. Most people believe that the gender attribution process is unequivocal; by contrast, Speer (2005) contends that such attributions are rarely trouble-free. When participants in her study were shown visual images of men and women engaging in non-traditionally gendered activities (men's ballet, women's rugby), they often displayed doubt and uncertainty.

Beliefs that there are two, and only two sexes, are not universally shared outside the west; other cultures have a more fluid sex/gender system and more accepting attitudes to gender variance. Amongst the Berdache North American Indians, for example, a third gender category exists which is neither male nor female; the hirjas of India, the kathoey of Thailand, the mak nyahs of Malaysia all eschew dichotomous gender categories. In Hinduism, not only are deities frequently ambiguous, but they can also change sex. In the Buddhist Vinaya text, four sex/gender categories have been identified (Winter and Udomsak, 2002). Transgender people in the west also do not fit into these gender categories and a dichotomous

system is unable to account for their experiences. Instead of shoehorn-
ing people into one or other of the two available sexes (Ekins and King,
1997), some argue that sex and gender are more accurately represented
by Kinsey-type continua (Feinberg, 2001).

Gender variance is well documented, possibly to a greater degree than
its prevalence might suggest (Ekins and King, 1997). Some claim that
Joan of Arc and Queen Elizabeth I were (what currently we would term
as) transgender. Representations are pervasive in both high and popular
culture including Shakespeare and children's pantomime; in transvestite
or drag performers such as Dame Edna Everidge, Eddie Izzard and Lily
Savage; and in film, theatre and literature including *Some Like it Hot*,
M Butterfly, *Billy Tipton*, *The Trumpet Player*, *Boys Don't Cry* and *The Crying
Game*. However, some characterisations infer that there is something
inherently deceptive in transgender which is reinforced by terms such as
female *impersonators*, *masquerade* and *drag*. Assumptions about deception
seem to be one of the ways heterosexism operates in relation to transgender. Transgender people are believed to be inherently duplicitous. The
notion of 'being real' is also used to gate-keep access to treatment: only
'real' transsexuals are eligible for surgery. Some argue that the increasing
numbers of transgender people prepared to go public about their identities including Jan Morris, Renee Richards, April Ashley, Dana International
(Eurovision song contest winner), Nadia Almada (winner of Big Brother
2004), Jenny Roberts, Parinya Charoenphol (Thai boxer) and Stephen
Whittle will contribute to increased public awareness and understanding of gender identity issues (Bullough, 2000; Dean et al., 2000).

The inclusion of transgender people is possibly the most controversial
in this chapter because the relationship between transgender and LGB
people has not been an easy one. The practice of drag has been dismissed
by some lesbian feminists as an insulting parody of women which
reinforces stereotypes in the wearing of high-heels and by an overly feminine appearance. Some gay men have also criticised the practice of drag
because of its association with effeminacy. Although transgender evokes
discomfort and disagreement, the greatest criticism has been reserved
for MtF (male to female – see below for an explanation) transsexuals.
Transsexuals in the UK are a relatively small group of people and of
them, a minority, identify as lesbian. Because few social spaces are available to them as transsexual lesbians, some join lesbian-only groups in
order to meet women. It is in these spaces that many disagreements sur-
face. Some lesbians (and many other people), reject MtF transwomen as
'real' women and refuse them access to lesbian groups. Some of the arguments used are that MtF transwomen have been socialised as males and

have no experience of oppression as women; they take up a disproportionate amount of time in lesbian groups by forcing their issues and,
because they retain male traits (such as expecting emotional support),
they do not feel the need to reciprocate. Moreover, they are said to dilute
or encroach on women-only space and because their concerns are different, transwomen should set up their own groups. While these arguments merit considerably more attention than is possible to devote to
them here, the debates adopt the biological and social essentialism that
characterised the early second-wave women's movement; in addition,
they presuppose that all women who are born female have an understanding of oppression. Instead, the following sections illustrate how the
dichotomous sex/gender system is interconnected with heterosexism.

Parallels with (some) lesbian experiences

While individual lesbians may never transgress the norms of appropriate gender behaviour, gender has been central to definitions of sexual
identity. There is a common misconception that to be lesbian or gay is
to want to be a member of the opposite sex. Women who are sexually
attracted to other women are believed to be defective women. Many lesbians (and gay men) find 'evidence' for their sexual identity in their
childhood preferences for climbing trees, playing with boys' toys and
other tomboyish behaviour. Non-conforming gender behaviour in children is said to be the most common element in the childhoods of lesbians and gay men (Bullough, 2000; Dean et al., 2000). Early sexologists
described lesbians as a 'third sex', 'inverts' or 'transvestite women'; they
were deemed to be 'men trapped in a woman's body'. The central character, Stephen Gordon, in Radclyffe Hall's lesbian classic *The Well of
Loneliness* epitomised this characterisation: in her personality, behaviour
and assumption of a male name. This tradition is continued by a number of contemporary lesbians who choose to masculinise their names
(e.g. Michelle/Mickey). Lesbian historians have uncovered evidence of
cross-dressed women in the eighteenth century who, conceiving their
love for another woman within a heterosexual paradigm, married their
female lover (Vicinus, 1993). In the 1950s, most lesbians had to choose
between the two available roles of butch and femme which were strin-
gently mandated by dress, role, behaviour and even personality traits.
Butches adopted highly stereotypical masculine behaviours – opening
doors, lighting cigarettes, courting and protecting – behaviours that so
called 'real men' were only seen to do in films (Faderman, 1992). One
famous butch lesbian, Louisa Dupont, about whom society gossiped
'She *walks* like a man, she *talks* like a man. God, she even *dresses* like

a man' was given the epithet *he-she* (Faderman, 1992: 170). 1950s lesbian-ism enforced (or was compelled to adopt) a rigid gender system which prescribed roles for butches and femmes. Despite this, an alternative term did exist – kiki – which suggested possibilities for being lesbian that did not conform to rigid gender binaries. Heterosexist models of gender identity and gender role may be adopted (or ascribed) by all those who transgress gender norms including lesbians and transgender people.[1]

By the 1980s, lesbians attempted to forge a third way between the pre-scriptive gender binaries adopted by earlier lesbians by challenging trad-itional heterosexist standards of what a woman should look (and be) like. An authentic lesbian self-presentation (looking dykey enough) was achieved by androgyny which frequently included short hair and finger-nails, jeans or dungarees and the rejection of feminine clothing. Androgyny is a gender category that is positioned outside of masculin-ity and femininity. Despite this, the term transgender notably excludes androgynous fashions in youth culture (Ekins and King, 1997). Lesbians also began to challenge gender expectations in terms of entering non-traditional occupations and in new ways of doing intimate relationships. These challenges to heteronormative gender appearance and behaviour may suggest possibilities for growing transgender movements.

There appear to be some parallels in the conceptual understandings about transgender people and those about lesbians and gay men. Early analysts tended to explain transgender behaviour either as a type of homosexuality or a flight from homosexuality (Bullough, 2000). Because of this misconception, many researchers included transgender people in their studies without discussion of their different needs (Terry, 1995). Transsexual people feel, like some lesbians have done, that they were born into the wrong body. Like lesbians and gay men, transgender people are said to be pathological or unhealthy because of their identities. One UK study suggested that there was a high incidence of displacement and separation in the childhoods of transsexual people (Di Ceglie et al., 2002); however, experience of the biological and psychological theories that have been used to explain the aetiology of homosexuality might suggest that we treat such perspectives with caution.

1. While there is continued discussion about butch/femme roles and appearance in lesbian relationships, the butch/femme attribution process seems far from unequivocal. For example, among our friends and acquaintances most people would probably describe my partner as butch and me as femme (these are, at times, hotly debated by the two of us). But in other circumstances where our heterosexuality is assumed (in restaurants, aeroplanes and so on) I am always the one who is addressed as sir.

There are, however, important differences between 'passing' as the opposite gender (and even in taking hormones) and undergoing sex reassignment surgery to physically alter the body. Transsexuals choose to surgically alter their bodies. There appear to be two main arguments that lesbian feminists have made about transsexuals. First, feminists have argued that transsexuals' desire for surgical procedures perpetuates a rigid gender system. The argument is made that transsexuals would not seek surgery if it were not for patriarchal oppression. Because of this, transsexuals are said to lack a political perspective and are marked out as distinct from other sexual minorities. By contrast to homosexuals, the aim of transsexuals is to leave their minority grouping behind in order to 'pass' as the opposite sex (Parsons, 2005). Rather than seeking a politicised identity, transsexuals are seen to desire to 'jump the sex/gender divide'; 'escape from their newly stigmatised identity'; and to finally 'pass as real men and women' (Parsons, 2005: 61). This process, whereby a transsexual alters the body to become a member of the opposite sex, does not leave intact the sex/gender system, as many would argue, but instead poses a fundamental challenge to our notions of what it means to be a woman or a man. Our 'natural attitude' is that gender is invariant: 'if you are female/male, you always were female/male and you always will be female/male' and there are no transfers from one gender to another (McKenna and Kessler, 2000: 12). By altering their physical bodies, transsexuals challenge these taken for granted assumptions. Transsexual activists argue that, rather than maintaining binary sex/gender categories, the lives and practices of transsexuals reveal the social construction of gender and are integral to the feminist project of challenging gender categories (Golden, 2000).

Second, many lesbian feminists, while supporting people's ability to make decisions about their own bodies, are uncomfortable with any surgical or hormonal alteration of the body to fit with cultural norms (Golden, 2000). The increasing trend of breast enlargement and facial reconstruction among non-transsexual women does not contribute to ending their oppression. Golden (2000) makes the point that it is similarly hard to see genital surgery or mastectomy as solutions to sex/gender dysphoria. While I found myself in agreement with her argument, she goes on to draw comparison with the principle of feminist opposition to female genital mutilation (FGM). This reminded me of the lessons (white) feminists needed to learn in allowing black feminists space to determine the agenda about FGM. Many African feminists have since spearheaded the campaign against FGM both in the UK and abroad. They wanted to articulate their concerns in their own voices. As a lesbian feminist, I do not understand the desire to undergo surgery, but nor do I assume that this desire is driven by a fundamentally conservative agenda. We need to make space for transsexual people: there is an absence of their own voices. The few accounts which are heard (usually in the mass media) are from people who regret the decision to undergo surgery. We need to hear from those who have made fulfilled lives following surgery, as well as look to possibilities that mean surgery is no longer the only available option.

The last decade has seen the increasing politicisation of the transgender movement and considerable progress has been made in their civil rights' claims (Munro, 2003). A landmark case in the European court in 1999 made it illegal to discriminate against someone on the basis of their transsexuality; this enables those who are transitioning to remain in their jobs. In 2003, the Gender Recognition Act enabled one's birth certificate to be changed and with it the right to marry and adopt a child with a partner of the opposite sex.

What is transgender?

The term transgender encompasses a wide range of social groupings including cross-dressers, drag queens and kings, intersexed people and transsexuals who have divergent interests and concerns. Initially, transgender was developed to describe people who transgress gender binaries without necessarily having surgery. There is some contention about its use; some transsexuals wish to claim the term because transsexuality concerns gender rather than sexuality (Munro, 2003). It should be noted here that feminists have suggested that both gender *and* sex are socially constructed categories (Kessler and McKenna, 2000). Some argue that any discussion of transgender people as a group is problematic because of the group's diversity (Meyer, 2001; Laird and Aston, 2003). Currently, most transgender individuals are either female to male (FtM) – sometimes called transmen – or male to female (MtF) – called transwomen (Dean et al., 2000). It is important to know that aspects of a person's gender and physical form can vary widely and be influenced by different factors (Lombardi, 2001); but because so little is known about transgender identities, definitions form a useful baseline of information (see Dean et al., 2000 for further consideration). Although these are presented as distinct categories, some suggest that MtF transsexuals often go through a period of cross-dressing before seeking surgery.

Transsexuals

Transsexuals are people who usually seek a range of medical interventions including hormone therapy, sex reassignment surgery, and speech and language therapy in order to achieve their need to live full time as members of the opposite sex. They are the group most likely to come into contact with a range of health professionals. Before clinical intervention is offered, the intending transitioner must live in the opposite gender for a year. This is known as the 'Real Life Test' which demonstrates their ability to integrate socially in this role. Internationally, treatment protocols are determined by recognised standards of care drawn up by the Harry Benjamin International Gender Dysphoria Association (HBIGDA) which are regularly updated. While some see them as gate-keeping access to treatment, others suggest they offer protection from inappropriate treatment or exploitation. Providers of health services regard the standards as authoritative, while many clients see them as restrictive (Lombardi, 2001).

Cross-dressers

Cross-dressers (transvestites) are people (primarily heterosexual men) who, although they dress in the clothing of the opposite sex, identify with their biological sex. People cross-dress for a number of reasons including social, emotional or erotic reasons. There may be different motivations between men who cross-dress and women who do so. Female to male cross-dressers have adopted male clothing for economic reasons – to gain employment as a man, to be accepted in a male role (the South Asian *Bandit Queen*) or to live openly with another woman.

Transgender

In addition to its use as an umbrella term, transgender also refers to people whose psychological self-identification is with the other sex. They alter their behaviour and appearance to conform to this perception, sometimes with the assistance of hormonal treatment. Some transgender people identify as both male and female, others as neither male nor female. Sometimes they retain the characteristics of both sexes (e.g. breasts and penis).

Intersex

Intersex describes people who are born with the physical characteristics of both sexes due to a naturally occurring combination of chromosomes, gonads and genitals (androgen insensitivity syndrome). Some undergo surgical procedures which remove the characteristics of one sex (usually the penis), but for some intersexed people their assigned gender does not match with their self-perception and in adolescence they may seek to undergo medical procedures to align their gender with their sex. Although they do not have ovaries and uteri, XY women develop as 'normal' females in their capacity for sexual response and sexual desire (Bullough, 2000).

Drag queens and kings

Drag queens and kings cross-dress to entertain, for personal satisfaction or to challenge gender stereotypes. The clothes of the opposite gender are worn for theatrical effect. Wearing drag differs from transvestism in that the cross-dresser usually seeks to pass as the opposite sex, whereas the drag queen or king mimics the opposite gender (Stewart, 1995). While drag queens have a long history, drag kings are a more recent social phenomenon.

Oppression of transgender people

The wearing of female clothes by men is usually an object of mirth or pity. Those who wish to surgically alter (those who disapprove use the term mutilate) their otherwise healthy bodies are considered deluded or apolitical. Many people do not accept that men can become women through surgery. Even in largely supportive articles there is an assumption that most post-operative transsexuals are dissatisfied with the results of their sex reassignment surgery (SRS) (Fee et al., 2003). Some warn of a loss of sexual feeling for both emotional and anatomical reasons and there appears to be a prurient interest in the details of the surgical operations as evidenced in recent media representations of the procedures. Gender variant boys appear to experience significantly more harassment than girls and this may be due to the fact that gender non-conformity is less acceptable in boys than in girls (Di Ceglie et al., 2002).

In order to achieve social integration, transgender people need to feel a sense of authenticity by 'passing' and being accepted by others. Medical professionals in gender identity clinics require a high degree of conformity to traditional gender roles in order to distinguish 'real' candidates (those who will subsequently receive surgery) from others. These assessments evaluate whether candidates are 'true women' in such areas as relationships with men, interest and caring for children and the capacity to work continuously in female occupations. One of the reasons (some) transsexuals may seem to conform to stereotyped female appearance and behaviour in the wearing of make-up and frilly, feminine clothes is that they have to prove to psychiatrists that they can pass as women.

The social status of transgender people

Although there are competing accounts about the social status of transgender people, most research (e.g. Winter and Udomsak, 2002) suggests that due to discrimination, even university graduates find it difficult to gain and sustain employment (although this situation may improve following recent legislative changes). Once transsexual people have transitioned, they are often forced into lower paid jobs. Rejection by their families and communities often means that they have had a disrupted childhood. School non-attendance is high among teenage transgender young people and results in fewer educational qualifications. As a consequence they experience unemployment, poverty and homelessness and a number turn to sex work as a means of earning a living (Nemoto et al., 2004).

What are transgender health issues?

There has been little large-scale research about the health and social care needs of transgender people and many studies are based on individual case histories. The experience of social and economic marginalisation places many transgender people at risk of alcohol abuse, depression, suicide and self-harm, substance abuse, HIV and a constant feeling of stress about gender and distress about body parts. Gender variance in young people represents a high suicide risk and indicates the importance of specialist treatment before, during and following puberty. Further, girls experience more depression and misery than boys (Di Ceglie et al., 2002).

MtF transgender people have the highest incidence of HIV infection of any risk group in San Francisco (Nemoto et al., 2004). Furthermore, there are ethnic differences in seroprevalence with African-Americans showing the highest rate. Among the 332 MtF transgender 'people of color' who took part in the study, those with HIV positive status were more likely than those without to report unprotected receptive anal intercourse and injection drug use in the past six months.

Access to health care

Transgender people represent an underserved community in need of comprehensive primary care (Feldman and Bockting, 2001). Those who wish to undergo SRS are subject to health authority quota systems which limit funded surgical procedures to one or two per year. Data suggest that approximately 1 per 30 000 adult males and 1 per 100 000 adult females seek SRS. *Press for Change* estimate that large numbers of transgender people are refused NHS treatment. They receive inadequate psychological counselling at overcrowded centres and after many years of hormone treatment, often find that surgery is denied them (retrieved 6 April 2005 from http://www.pfc.org.uk).

Failure to distinguish gender identity from sexual identity means that many health professionals assume that transgender patients have the same health needs as LGB (Finlon, 2002). Health professionals are said to hold widely polarised views of transsexualism and gender dysphoria, ranging from strong moral disapproval to considerable empathy. Lack of knowledge means, for example, that FtM individuals are rarely included in breast screening programmes despite continuing risk for those who have experienced female pubertal breast development unless all their breast tissue has been removed (Eyler and Whittle, 2001). Physical examinations and screening tests should be offered to patients on the basis of the organs present rather than their perceived gender (Feldman and Bockting, 2001). Intersexed people have rarely received a diagnosis or information about their chromosomal characteristics and surgery received as a child.

Discrimination against transgender people has included the refusal of care such as smear tests, breaches of their confidentiality and the practice of placing transsexual women who have completed sex reassignment surgery on male wards. Feinberg describes being refused care by an emergency room physician:

> Five years ago, while battling an undiagnosed case of bacterial endocarditis, I was refused care at a Jersey City emergency room. After the physician who examined me discovered that I am female-bodied, he ordered me out of the emergency room despite the fact that my temperature was above 104 Fahrenheit. He said I had a fever 'because you are a very troubled person'. (Feinberg, 2001: 897)

These experiences may make many transgender people reluctant to seek health care. In the US, the Gay and Lesbian Medical Association has issued guidelines for creating a safe clinical environment for lesbian, gay, bisexual, transgender and intersex patients in order to improve access to quality care. Transgender women may also be uncomfortable in disclosing their gender history to providers (Nemoto et al., 2005). Intersex women report being repeatedly asked about their last period and their contraceptive use; some are given smears (although they do not have a cervix).

Mental health

In order for transsexual people to gain access to SRS, they need to be assessed as meeting one of the four criteria in the *Diagnostic and Statistical Manual of Mental Disorders (DSM-IV)*. The *DSM-IV* defines gender identity disorder (GID) as a strong and persistent cross gender identification which is the desire to be, or the insistence one is, of the other sex and persistent discomfort about one's assigned sex or a sense of inappropriateness of the gender role of that sex. In order to make a diagnosis, there must be evidence of clinically significant distress or impairment in social, occupational or other important areas of functioning. Although being transsexual does not constitute a mental disorder under the *DSM-IV*, in order to gain access to sex reassignment surgery, transsexual people must meet its criteria. The criteria medicalise transsexual identities. Some advocates argue for a declassification of GID; others argue for maintaining the classification because the inclusion of GID in the *DSM–IV* may allow for insurance reimbursement (in the US) and treatment for transsexual people (Dean et al., 2000).

The inclusion of transgender issues in the health and social care needs agenda is uneven. A major setback was the failure to include transgender issues in the US public health strategy document *Healthy People 2010* (Meyer, 2001). In a review of twenty years of public health research between 1980 and 1999, Boehmer (2002) found that the proportion of articles on transgender health decreased by 21 per cent and much of the research is pathology focused. In the UK, while there has been an upsurge of research and activist commitment to the health and social care needs of sexual minorities (e.g. Pringle, 2003; Scott et al., 2004), there needs to be inclusion of transgender people in studies as well as separate consideration of their health and social care needs.

Working class lesbians, bisexuals and gay men

Historical perspectives

There is less research specifically about class than about any other of the LGB identities; working class LGB are among the least represented in studies. This appears to be the case across the diverse range of LGB communities; even in research among black same-sex communities, black working class LGB are under-represented (Battle et al., 2002). There are no social groups with LGB working class affiliations and few public organisations with an explicit LGB working class membership. Even among trade unions, the traditional institution of the working classes, there is strongest representation by the middle classes on LGB caucuses. Working class LGB occupy different social spaces and may not be accessible through methods frequently used to recruit LGB to studies: snowballing is one technique that proved less effective in sampling working class lesbians (Taylor, 2005). In the contemporary social climate, LGB are overwhelmingly believed to be middle class. This assumption was recently articulated in a radio interview with MP Joe Ashton in which it was allegedly reported that 'there are no lesbians in Barnsley'. The remark appears to have been made to disassociate the working class from lesbianism.

This lack of a public profile has not always been the case; in the 1950s and 1960s, bars were the most visible institution associated with working class LGB. Faderman (1992) documents a vibrant, working class, lesbian social history in which bars formed an important cultural space and butch/femme roles characterised many of the relationships. Not all butch/femme lesbians are working class, nor do all working class lesbians adopt butch/femme identities. However, in many of the personal accounts of working class lesbian lives – where much of the social history is recorded – a butch or femme identity is described. Butches were known by their appearances, femmes by their choices. Working class lesbians of the 1950s and 1960s were frontline warriors against heterosexist oppression. It was predominantly working class LGB who precipitated the 1969 Stonewall rebellion, which launched the Gay Liberation Movement, by fighting back against a police raid.

In the 1970s a new generation of women came out as lesbians; they were more likely to be educated and middle class. The existence of butch/femme lesbian sub-cultures was seen to compromise the status and political understandings of middle class lesbians who adopted an androgynous appearance. Butch/femme lifestyles were often dismissed as reactionary and non-feminist; they were sometimes vilified because they seemed to be derivative of heterosexual values and relationships. Yet talk about class was remarkably absent from discussions in lesbian movements, except as a synonym for poverty (Plumb, 1997). Some activists argue that the lesbian-feminist cultural revolution of the 1970s left a gap in lesbian heritage by denying the experiences of those lesbians who had preceded them.

Class oppression

Class is notoriously resistant to cultural categorisation. Plumb (1997) argues that class is about socialisation, your sense of entitlement, how you feel about yourself and the world around you. Class places limits on people's life opportunities. UK studies have tended to rely on occupation-based measures, like the registrar general's classification, to measure class. But class can be signified by (among other things) housing type and tenure, school attended, own, or parental, qualifications, household income, car ownership or accent. There are also lifestyle factors associated with class, such as exercise and leisure activities, eating habits, smoking, family and kinship networks, values and attitudes. Although class is a white western construct, the social inequalities that class often acts as shorthand for, are also experienced by black people.

In one of the few studies of working class lesbian identities, McDermott (2004) draws upon Bourdieu's concepts of linguistic capital and habitus to explore lesbians' classed positions. She notes that the linguistic ease and communicative competence of the middle class distinguish them from working class lesbians. She draws attention to the scarcity of positive class discourses; in many, the working class are depicted as deviant and lacking in self-control. These discourses echo those which pathologised homosexuality. Habitus mediates our interaction with the social world; the personal accounts of working class lesbians are characterised by a lack of confidence, self-worth and expectation.

Access to health and social care

There is an established tradition of health inequalities research which has revealed, for example, stark differences in average age of death by social class and area of residence: working class men in Glasgow and Manchester may have up to five years' reduced life expectancy in comparison to a middle class man living in the south east. The classic *Black Report* (1979) provided evidence of a range of health and health care inequalities. Working class people tended to have shorter consultations with their GP than middle class patients and discussed fewer problems. Even when working class patients had been registered for a longer period with their GP practice, doctors had less knowledge about their personal and domestic circumstances; working class patients were also less likely to be visited by their GP in hospital (Townsend and Davidson, 1979). Working class women are likely to be at increased risk of cervical cancer in comparison to middle class women, but they are less likely to have attended for a smear test (Townsend and Davidson, 1979). These issues may be compounded for working class lesbians.

There is no research (that I have been able to find) about working class LGBT access to health and social care. Marj Plumb (1997), a leading figure in lesbian health advocacy, provides one of the few discussions. Despite having come out to her health care workers fifteen years previously, their heterosexist assumptions still limited her access to care. Moreover, as a butch working class lesbian, some gynaecological procedures such as smear tests and mammograms were especially uncomfortable.

LGB people living in rural communities

Living in a rural area may be a key social determinant in the health and social care needs of LGB communities. Although lesbians, gay men, bisexual and transgender people who live in rural areas are not oppressed in terms of their identity, they are likely to experience difficulties in accessing appropriate services. While many LGB people have relocated to urban areas, LGB people who work in rural industries, such as farming, are unable to do so. People who live in rural areas tend to be more socially conservative than those who live in cities; consequently, LGB people who live in rural areas may face increased levels of heterosexism. They are likely to have reduced access to social support groups or have to travel long distances to access them; they are more likely to be isolated; they are likely to fear breaches of their confidentiality in smaller communities (Tiemann et al., 1998); and there may be fewer service providers with knowledge or expertise in LGB needs.

Towards inclusive health and social care agendas

In reviewing the literature for this chapter, it is evident that there is a need for future research. Studies are needed among younger (i.e. under 18) LGBT, and on how participation in LGBT social groups can support identity formation and the coming out process. There is little UK research on or with black lesbians and gay men, in particular about their intimate relationships and their access to health and social care. Finally, while there is a relatively large body of work on transgender issues, most of it is clinical or pathology focused, and there is little about their social and health care needs.

The interlocking nature of oppression has been recognised for more than three decades; paradoxically, 'academics, policy makers and activists have a long tradition of ignoring the intersections and interactions between these social divisions' (Beckett and Macey, 2001: 309). This chapter aimed to address this gap in the literature and illustrate the heterogeneity of LGBT people's needs; there is not one single LGBT experience and heterosexism has different effects in relation to different identities. Importantly, many LGBT people have multiple identities: for example, they may be black, working class and transgender. There is growing recognition that knowledge about intersecting identities is important to inform the work of the new single equality body (see Chapter 9), which brings together six of the identities discussed here, and to influence policy development.

4
Conducting Research among LGB Communities

Methodological challenges in LGB health and social care research

Two methodological challenges have dominated thinking in research among LGB communities. The first concerns conceptual issues – who is a lesbian or a gay man? Is being LGB determined by sexual behaviour, attraction or political identification as a lesbian or gay man? The chosen definition will determine who will take part in a study. Can someone be LGB if they have never engaged in same-sex sexual behaviour? While heterosexuality is not defined by sexual activity, being lesbian, gay or bisexual commonly is so defined. Yet many LGB will be excluded by a definition that relies on sexual behaviour; young LGB may be attracted to someone of the same sex, but have not acted on that desire. In addition, celibate gay men pose a challenge to dominant conceptions of gay male identities. Yet for some, it is the basis of their acceptance as clergy within the Anglican Church.

The second challenge is a sampling issue: how are the diverse communities recruited to research? Making contact with diverse communities, as Chapter 3 illustrated, requires different sampling frames because groups have a range of forms of social association and are likely to be less accessible through membership lists of social organisations or other semi-formal means of contact. Recently, researchers have begun to reconceptualise LGBT identities, to rethink their sampling strategies and make additional efforts to reach these 'hidden' populations. This chapter considers the ways lesbians and gay men have been defined; sampling issues in LGB research; and developments in LGB non-probability research.

Defining lesbians and gay men

Decisions about who should be included in research are often determined by the topic under investigation; defining who is going to take part is the first step in recruiting participants. In the case of a study about the health of post-menopausal women, the definition might be relatively clear-cut: those eligible to take part could be identified as women aged 50–79. Many researchers would consider the definition unproblematic; however, it might exclude women who experienced an early menopause, women who had never had a menstrual cycle and transgender women. Researchers among LGB communities have also advocated 'singular and unambiguous' definitions (Sell and Petrulio, 1996: 34); however, these tend to homogenise LGB identities. There is no consensus among researchers about what it means to be a lesbian or a gay man because definitions are reflective of wider social debates and the language used has changed over time and differs between cultural groups. When Sell and Petrulio (1996) conducted a review of LGB research, most studies did not conceptually define the population nor describe the settings used to select participants. There have been a range of ways that researchers have used to define lesbians and gay men and these are considered below.

The use of setting to define participants

In the early twentieth century, the term 'homosexual' was widely used to denote both men and women; however, its use was not neutral for it implied deviance, abnormality and sin. Such preconceptions meant that researchers saw nothing problematic in recruiting LGB people who were incarcerated in institutions, mainly prisons or psychiatric hospitals. Not surprisingly, they were found to be criminally inclined or emotionally disturbed. Study participants who were recruited from clinical, or other such settings, were unlikely to be representative of LGB communities as a whole. By the mid-1960s, researchers were experimenting with other methods of gaining access to LGB people; one of the most common approaches was to recruit participants through gay bars. Bars represented one of the most important social gathering spaces for lesbians and gay men when few other public outlets were available to them. They provided one of the few ways by which researchers could gain access to lesbian and gay populations. In many of these studies, researchers did not ask the simple question 'are you homosexual?' [sic], but instead behaved as 'spies in public rendezvous' and covertly included them in studies (De Cecco, 1981: 58). More often than not, participants' sexual identity was simply assumed: potential participants were deemed to be lesbian or gay because of the setting in which they were recruited. The socio-demographic characteristics of lesbians and gay men sampled from a gay bar may be untypical of the population as a whole.

Rejecting the use of clinical populations, a number of researchers began to consider alternative methods for recruiting participants. One of the most enduring has been the use of social organisations such as the Minorities Research Group in the UK or the Mattachine Society and the Daughters of Bilitis in the US. June Hopkins' UK study (1969) is an early example of this method which included a sample of 48 participants of equal numbers of lesbian and heterosexual women. Hopkins' use of the Kinsey (1953) scale demonstrated an early commitment to conceptual definitions of lesbian identity.

The Kinsey scale and the sexual identity continuum

Kinsey and colleagues (1953) were among the first to propose that homosexuality exists along a continuum; research respondents were placed, depending on their sexual history and psychosexual responses, along a scale of 0–6 where zero was entirely heterosexual and 6 entirely homosexual. Even though the study was concerned with sexual behaviour, an individual could receive a rating on the scale even if he or she had no overt heterosexual or homosexual experience (Kinsey et al., 1953: 470). The notion of a homosexual continuum has been used to widen the scope for inclusion of a greater number of lesbians and gay men in research. Kinsey's study was widely credited with challenging beliefs about the prevalence of same-sex sexual behaviour. It was also ground-breaking because sexual identity was linked not only to sexual behaviour, but also to identity and/or desire. The continuum is useful in its social inclusivity: one of his research aims was to show that same-sex sexual behaviour was more prevalent than previously imagined. Because his findings suggested that homosexuality was commonly practised, it could not be considered abnormal. The Kinsey scale is a mechanism for operationally identifying research participants which is used by current researchers. It includes two dimensions of sexual identity – desire and behaviour – and allows participants some control over the way they are defined. While Kinsey's scale for defining homosexuality continues to be used by lesbian, gay and bisexual researchers, his sampling methods attracted considerable controversy. Moreover, the size of his sample – 11 240 participants – has been only infrequently achieved in subsequent research.

Sexual exclusivity as a criterion for definition

The newly emerging women's movement sparked debates about the meanings of lesbianism. Partly out of a developing separatist agenda, one of the definitions proposed a sexual exclusivity criterion: you were lesbian only if you did not currently have sex with men. While the definition may have had the benefit of differentiating lesbians from heterosexual women, the disadvantages included its premise upon absent behaviour; moreover, it was unclear how long this period of sexual exclusivity should be. The criterion was rather rigidly applied during the early debates on HIV/ AIDS when researchers at the US Center for Disease Control made the – now infamous – decision (see Plumb, 2001) to categorise as lesbian only those women who had had sex exclusively with women in the previous 13 years (Chu et al., 1990). The findings were controversial; many argued that the research excluded large numbers of women who, although they self-identified as lesbian, had had sex with men during the specified period. The study was influential in constructing assumptions that lesbians were not at risk of HIV based on beliefs that lesbians did not have sex with men. The study illustrates the inter-relation of topic and conceptual definitions. Clarity about their topic of investigation and how it related to definitions may have averted some of the criticisms. If the aim was to investigate whether lesbian sex was a transmission route for HIV, then sexual behaviour with women is relevant; sexual behaviour with men (irrespective of lesbian identity) is not. On the other hand, if the research was concerned about lesbians' risk of HIV, then lesbian identities needed to be broadly defined. Overly prescriptive definitions, even when they reflect current debates, may not be helpful in selecting participants for study.

Self-definition as a criterion

Categorisation by the research team in the above example was also controversial because it located the power to define – and thus to include or exclude someone from research – with the researcher rather than study participants. Many writers believed that identities should not be assigned by others but only self-reported: you are only lesbian if you say you are (Faderman, 1992). The move in research to self-reporting as a method paralleled developments in lesbian and gay activism. Many lesbians and gay men publicly identified themselves so that a declared and discrete identity could be organised around. Self-naming meant that the overarching feature of lesbian or gay identity was not solely determined by a man or woman's sexual behaviour and it allowed for a range of inclusions built on people's own understandings. Self-identification has been the most frequent method used to define lesbians and gay men. Survey researchers using this conceptual definition will usually include a statement which clarifies who potential participants might be (e.g. Fish, 2002).

Self-identification as a lesbian or gay man is particularly relevant for studies which investigate experiences of heterosexism or research about levels of disclosure and non-disclosure. For example, a woman – who has sex with women, but who does not identify as lesbian – would be unable to reflect on the way a health professional reacts to her lesbian identity.

A limitation of self-identification, however, is that people's understandings differ widely. A woman can have sex with women and men and define herself as lesbian, bisexual, heterosexual or even reject a 'label'. On the other hand, some women have never had sex with another woman, but identify as lesbian. The term lesbian has not been universally accepted among lesbians themselves: older lesbians sometimes have preferred to use 'gay woman' to describe themselves while some black women have felt that the word 'lesbian' marginalised their experiences because of its origins in the Greek island of Lesbos. In the words of Elaine, a black woman involved in the Women's Movement, who had a longstanding partnership with another woman: 'I didn't like the word lesbian. Because I wasn't white, I didn't wear dungarees, I didn't go to Greenham Common so I couldn't have been one' (Fish, 1993: 33). There have been a number of challenges to a politics of identity because it (potentially) excluded growing numbers of lesbians who were black, disabled and working class. Self-reported identities obscured these differences in meanings and they depended upon the self-conscious adoption of a lesbian or gay identity. Furthermore, self-reported identity tends to include those who are most confident, visible and highly affiliated with lesbian and gay communities.

Definitions based on sexual behaviours

Public health concerns, especially over HIV and other STIs, have also determined how homosexuality is defined. The two largest studies to be conducted in the early 1990s were driven by this agenda and their focus was primarily sexual behaviour (Laumann et al., 1994; Wellings et al., 1994). Because such studies needed to include the diverse range of men who have same-sex partners, researchers looked for ways to make definitions inclusive. One strategy has been to prioritise sexual behaviour (above identity) and the term 'gay man' (especially) has been replaced in some studies by 'men who have sex with men' (MSM) (Hickson et al., 1998). This is because not all men who engage in sex with other men identify themselves as gay, especially married men. Moreover, there are cultural differences about meanings; in some communities the term 'gay' is applied only to the passive partner (although this might assume rigidly ascribed sexual practices). MSM, as definition, has been a useful means of including men from black communities. The turn in research among LGB communities

is towards definitions which facilitate inclusion and allow research participants to identify themselves along a continuum rather than a narrowly
prescribed category (see Chapter 9 for an alternative perspective on the
use of MSM).

Different dimensions of same-sex identity

In the light of these difficulties about terminology and meanings,
researchers (Solarz, 1999) have looked to develop definitions that are more
inclusive of women and men who exhibit differing degrees of same-sex
behaviour, desire or identity in combinations that vary between individuals. Defining the population solely by its sexual behaviour is likely
to exclude people who identify as gay even though they have not had
any same-sex sexual experience. In a US national study of sexual behaviour, Laumann et al. (1994) identified lesbians and gay men by three criteria of desire, behaviour and identity. Their study was particularly valuable
for demonstrating the effect of definition upon the sample recruited: the
number of lesbians or gay men in a sample varies according to the definition used. Of the 143 men in the study, more were identified by desire
(44 per cent) than by behaviour (24 per cent) or identity (2 per cent).
Similarly, in a study by Brogan et al. (2001) the sample contained 90 lesbians if the criterion of self-reported identity was used, while 115 participants were included by current sexual activity and identity.

The current challenge in research among LGB communities is to design
strategies which encourage participation from diverse communities. One
such strategy has been to widen notions of sexual identity by using the
term 'non-heterosexual' (Heaphy et al., 2003). This avoids categorising
people by behaviour or identity, but its meaning may not be widely understood. Another innovation, devised by Morris and Rothblum (1999),
was in a study which examined the degree to which women are distributed on five aspects of lesbian sexuality and the coming out process.
These five aspects were: (a) sexual orientation (numerical rating of sexual identity from exclusively lesbian to exclusively heterosexual); (b) years
out (length of time of self-identity as lesbian or bisexual); (c) outness
(amount of disclosure to others); (d) sexual experience (proportion of
relationships with women); (e) lesbian activities (extent of participation
in lesbian community events). The research investigated whether there
were associations between number of years out; numbers of people to
whom one had disclosed; number of sexual experiences with women;
the frequency of attendance at lesbian-only events; and self-identification
as lesbian. Being lesbian was not a homogeneous experience: African-
American women who self-defined as lesbian were most likely to have

had sexual experiences with women; they were also more likely to be out and to participate in lesbian activities. The research confounded a widespread assumption, namely that white lesbians were more likely to be identified on these dimensions. By contrast, among white lesbians, there was no association between the length of time they had been out and the number of people they had disclosed to.

Concluding remarks about defining lesbians, gay men and bisexuals

Some researchers have proposed the adoption of universal definitions of same-sex identities (e.g. Sell and Petrulio, 1996). As I have endeavoured to show, the terms used and the meanings invested in sexual identity have changed over time. Decisions about whether to include a transgender lesbian in a study about lesbian health, is a theoretical matter first. Researchers should clarify their definition and their reasons for using it and these will be related to the topic and the research aims. Moreover, the current priority is towards social diversity because many previous studies have excluded those who are most marginalised. Research among lesbians, gay men and bisexuals has often failed to include LGB people under the age of 20 (excepting university students) and over the age of 50; black communities; those who are unemployed, disabled, working class, transgender or bisexual; those living in rural communities; and those who are less 'out' to others. Clarity about potential participants is useful for informing a sampling frame to recruit them.

Sampling issues in LGB communities

Research conducted among lesbian and gay communities has come under sustained criticism for failing to use sufficiently rigorous sampling methods. Studies have frequently produced samples which are predominantly white, middle class, well-educated and the participants are aged between 25 and 40 years old. A major challenge to researchers then is said to be the construction of representative samples by the use of probability sampling (often known as random sampling) (Solarz, 1999). Probability sampling, that is, sampling where every member of a clearly specified population has an equal chance of being selected, is generally seen to be the scientifically acceptable way to construct a sample. Probability sampling contributes to the rigour and validity of the research conducted. By selecting research participants through random methods, researchers are able to say that the characteristics found in the sample, such as health care behaviours, can be generalised to the population as a whole. If a sampling frame is badly constructed, it is unlikely to be able to represent the socio-demographics of the target population. Examples drawn from mainstream research of voting intentions – a visible means of demonstrating whether a sample was representative – serve to illustrate this issue. The *Literary Digest* poll, which drew its sample from lists of telephone ownership and car registrations, incorrectly predicted the 1936 US presidential election (despite canvassing the views of almost two million potential voters), because Republican voters were more likely to have telephones and cars than were Democrats. Similarly, opinion polls on the eve of the British general election of 1992 forecast a Labour victory – which a day later proved spectacularly wrong – because a number of people (assumed to be Labour voters) had removed themselves from the Electoral Register (and were thus not eligible to vote) in protest at the Poll Tax which had been newly introduced by the Conservatives. In order to make an accurate prediction (in this case of voting intentions) there needs to be a good match between the sample and the population it is designed to represent and these examples highlight that *what kinds of people* are selected is as important as *how many*. Furthermore, survey researchers typically have access to a range of data about their target population which enables them to assess the degree to which their sample is reflective of it. Because data about people living in same-sex relationships were only included in the census for the first time in 2001, we do not know with certainty how many lesbians and gay men live in the UK, nor how many of them live alone, what jobs they hold or how their ages are distributed. It is, then, difficult to state the relationship between an achieved sample and the LGB population in the UK as a whole.

Limitations of probability research

While non-probability research has been criticised for its lack of scientific rigour, probability methods have not been similarly examined for their ability to sample among same-sex communities. There are six issues surrounding the use of random methods in LGB research, these are: (i) refusals to participate; (ii) non-disclosure; (iii) the size of the sample; (iv) costs of research; (v) the composition of the sample; (vi) concepts and terminology in non-probability sampling. These are considered in turn below.

(i) Refusals to participate

Probability researchers typically use the Electoral Register or the Postcode Address File as sampling frames for UK-based research (Fish, 2000). Neither of these sampling frames, however, identifies lesbians and gay men, and researchers must sample the whole population in order to obtain a sub-sample of lesbians and gay men. One of the problems facing probability researchers is not the issue of *selecting* lesbian, gay and bisexual participants to a study, but of *including* them. In the early 1990s, two national surveys of sexual behaviour were conducted in the US and in the UK and as they used probability methods, the researchers claimed to have produced a representative sample of lesbians and gay men on this basis alone.

In any survey there will be a refusal rate (i.e. participants decline to take part in a study) of between 25 and 35 per cent (Smith, 2002). According to Laumann et al. (1994), the missing 25 per cent pose a serious problem for the reliability and validity of a survey if those people who refuse to participate differ in a systematic way from those who do participate. The US National Health and Social Life Survey (NHSLS) (Laumann et al., 1994) produced a sample in which only 0.7 per cent of participants (150 women) were located on the lesbian continuum (of desire, behaviour or identity). While the authors acknowledge that no other single number in their study would attract greater public interest, they do not account for any possible effects of the topic under investigation (the epidemiology of HIV/AIDS) upon decisions to participate. In discussion of the study's response rate, they highlight a problem frequently encountered by interviewers where a number of potential participants did not think that AIDS affected them and therefore that 'information about their sex life would be of little use' (Laumann et al., 1994: 55). Yet they fail to discuss the effect of this perception upon the participation of lesbians. In the early 1990s, lesbians were frequently described as being at low risk for HIV/AIDS (Richardson, 1994) and it may be that a greater proportion of lesbians than any other group decided not to participate in a study that appeared to have little relevance to them.

Two large-scale studies of sexual behaviour – the US NHSLS and the UK National Survey of Sexual Attitudes and Lifestyles (NATSAL 1990) (Wellings et al., 1994) – were the first national probability surveys to include a sub-sample of lesbians, gay men and bisexuals. Both were influential in providing estimates for the LGB population in their respective countries (see Chapter 5).

Wellings et al. (1994) contended that their survey was authoritative because, unlike volunteer samples, whose participants may self-select, a random sample reduces the likelihood of this occurring. While the demographic characteristics of those who declined to participate in NATSAL (which was also about the epidemiology of AIDS) are not known, there is some evidence to suggest that gay men were reluctant to take part. A study of 500 gay men by Project Sigma asked whether they would participate in NATSAL 1990. Half of them said they would refuse and a further third said they would take part, but hide the fact they were gay (Stanley, 1995).

(ii) Non-disclosure

Although refusals are not unique to lesbian and gay potential participants, lesbians and gay men can refuse to participate in unique ways. They can refuse to *come out* in a study by 'falsely saying' they are heterosexual (Bradford et al., 1997) or by declining to answer questions about sexual identity. In one of the largest studies of older women's health which included details about sexual orientation, lesbians comprised 0.6 per cent (N = 573 of 93 311) of the sample (Valanis et al., 2000). However, a further 2696 women (2.8 per cent) in the sample declined to answer questions about sexual identity – the authors feared they were more likely to be lesbians – and were excluded from the study because of the missing data. In a telephone survey, similar proportions of women failed to disclose their sexual identity (Meyer et al., 2002). Although we do not know whether lesbians are more likely to hide their sexual orientation than heterosexual women, a telephone survey found that women were much more likely to disclose their heterosexuality than they were to identify as lesbian (Bradford et al., 1997). Thirty-two (6 per cent) women refused to answer the question and while the researchers did not know who these women were, in such a context it is hard to see why a heterosexual woman would refuse to identify herself (although see Chapter 1 for discussion) because there is mainly social benefit not social stigma associated with heterosexuality. The decision to disclose as lesbian or heterosexual is not symmetrical. By identifying as lesbian, a woman adopts a politicised identity. Moreover, some lesbians and gay men may choose to hide their sexual identity – and be more practised at it – because they fear ostracism from their family or social disapproval. The refusal to come out is possibly the biggest challenge facing researchers who have looked to new ways of facilitating disclosure.

(iii) The size of the sample

Probability sampling methods typically produce very small sub-samples of the LGB population. For example, in the US NHSLS (Laumann et al., 1994) only 23 (out of a total of 1749 women) self-identified as lesbian (on all three dimensions) while 31 (out of 10 942) did so in the NATSAL 1990 survey. Judgements about a representative sample achieved through probability sampling cannot be made on the basis of such low numbers. Yet while both research teams acknowledged that their sample was too small to consider variation in relation to ethnicity (even though they over-sampled among black communities), no similar caveats are made about sexual identity. Thirty-one women could only be said to represent UK lesbians in terms of age, 'race', class, disability, education, employment and geographic location if assumptions are made that lesbian communities are particularly homogeneous.

One might expect that subsequent research using probability methods would confirm earlier findings about the size of LGB populations. This has not been the case; the same survey (NATSAL 2000) conducted a decade later found an increase from 3.6 per cent in 1990 to 5.4 per cent in 2000 in the number of men who reported same-sex partnerships (Johnson et al., 2001). The greatest difference, however, was among women reporting female same-sex partners: the proportions more than doubled from 1.8 per cent in 1990 to 4.9 per cent in 2000. It does not seem likely that people remembered behaviours they had forgotten previously or that more people now identify as LGB. Johnson et al. (2001) argue that these changes result from improved survey methodology: CASI – a form of computer-assisted interviewing which allows participants to record their own responses to sensitive questions and preserves their anonymity. The increase may also be due to a greater willingness to report same-sex behaviour and more tolerant social attitudes. It indicates that improvements are needed in order to randomly sample among LGB communities and the prevailing social and political climate may have an impact on people's willingness to take part in research. Far from having 'settled' (Laumann et al., 1994: 286) the matter of the prevalence of homosexuality, these two studies appear to have opened the possibilities for further debate. The social and political climate has changed dramatically since NATSAL 2000 was conducted and these changing attitudes have been reflected in a raft of legislative reforms (see Appendix A).

(iv) Costs of research

Because there is no census-based sampling frame of the LGB population researchers must sample the population in general – the majority of whom are heterosexual – in order to obtain a sub-sample of LGB. The NHSLS and NATSAL both used survey interviews because they generally secure a higher response rate (approximately 75 per cent) than other methods. The NHSLS team acknowledged that high-quality research is an expensive operation and provided details of the costs of their study: $450 per completed interview and with a sample of 3432 the overall costs amounted to over $1.5 million. Postal questionnaires are a cheaper alternative, but they tend to achieve a lower response rate. Working on the assumption that an acceptable return rate is 50 per cent of mailed questionnaires, it would be necessary to mail out 20 000 questionnaires to achieve a sample of 10 000 heterosexual and lesbian women. Such a large sample would be needed in order to achieve a sufficiently large sub-sample to consider socio-demographic diversity. If lesbians represent 3–5 per cent of the total female population this would achieve a sub-sample of 300 to 500 lesbians (many purposive surveys recruit samples of 500 or more). The costs of managing a survey of this size, however, including administrative support, stationery, printing, postage, reminder mailings and incentives for reluctant responders (the latter two are typically used to bring the response rate up to acceptable levels) mean that probability methods are out of the reach of most researchers among LGB populations. In addition, these methods of encouraging reluctant respondents may not be effective given the nature of LGB refusals. Reminder mailings are a potential threat to privacy and anonymity and might not be effective in the light of one survey's findings (Fish, 2002) that a small number of respondents expressed concern at the area digits of their postcode (the final digits giving their street location were not requested) being known to the researcher. It is unlikely that a £10 gift token would encourage a respondent to participate in a survey where s/he had previously declined on the basis of anonymity, rather than not having got round to completing it. Funding does remain an obstacle: many lesbian health researchers have struggled with the difficulties in accessing research funds and speak of their experience of doing research on a 'shoe-string budget' (Fish, 1999).

(v) The composition of the sample

A compelling reason to support the use of probability sampling among LGB populations is their potential for achieving a sample that better represents the diversity of lesbian and gay communities. However, when Martin and Dean (1993) compared the demographics of their study, which used non-probability methods, to the results of studies using random sampling techniques – one of which was random digit-dialling (RDD) – they found that the composition of the three samples were broadly similar with regard to 'race', age and being 'out' of the closet. Education was the characteristic on which their New York City sample appeared to contrast most strongly with the two probability San Francisco samples. In Martin and Dean's (1993) study, 77 per cent had completed a four-year college degree, while in the San Francisco samples just over half had done so. Some of the large-scale studies using probability methods have failed to identify the demographic composition of their sample and thus it is impossible to tell whether they too over-represent LGB who are white, middle class and highly educated. Ethnicity in NATSAL 1990 was 95 per cent white – a larger proportion than that achieved by non-random methods (Fish, 2002).

(vi) Concepts and meanings in probability sampling

Although the NHSLS developed the notion of inter-related aspects of sexual identity, Laumann et al. (1994) paid most attention to sexual behaviour because it seemed to be one of the least ambiguous elements of sexual identity in general. However, they go on to acknowledge the over-simplification inherent in an exclusively behavioural approach, because of the widely divergent meanings of a given sexual act to participants. The study serves to illustrate some of the complexities in concepts and terminology about sex. Because it was a probability study of the whole population – heterosexual and homosexual – the phrasing of the questions needed to be understood by, and applicable to, all respondents. For example, many of the questions about sexual behaviour did not use language which assumed an opposite-sex partner. However, it is not simply sufficient to neutralise the gender of the sex partner in designing questions about sexual behaviour, but to rethink all of the meanings attached to sex. This is exemplified by the lead-in question to the section on sexual activity in the NHSLS which is prefaced by this introduction:

> Now I am going to be asking some questions about your sexual activity during the last 12 months. People mean different things by 'sex' or 'sexual activity' but in answering questions, we need everyone to use the *same definition*. Here by 'sex' or 'sexual activity' we mean any mutually voluntary activity with another person that involves *genital* contact and sexual excitement or arousal, that is, feeling really turned on even if *intercourse* or orgasm did not occur. (Laumann 1994: 622 emphasis added)

The implicit heterosexism of the question lies in the assumption that the same definition is possible for both homosexuals and heterosexuals: it is more likely to be the one that most represents the dominant sexual experience – heterosexuality. The question also assumes that lesbian sex mimics heterosexual sex and that the genital organs are the only (or main) site of sexual activity (such a definition is likely to be problematic for some heterosexual women also). Perhaps one of the most contested debates about lesbian experience – from sex radicals to lesbian feminist positions on sex and which some have characterised as the lesbian sex wars – is about lesbians' sexual behaviour. When Creith (1996: 66) asked participants in the Lesbian Sex Survey 'what would have to happen between you and another woman for you to call it sex' many lesbians did refer specifically to genital contact. But many others included a wide range of behaviour that they described as sex, including: anything that got me wet; anything that made me feel vulnerable; for us both to agree it was sex; any expression of desire – there isn't for me one act which means it's sex we're having; an activity in which one or both women try to bring the other to the point of orgasm; not necessarily physical: mind sex, verbal sex; I don't believe that sex necessarily has to be genital, hence caressing and stroking of the whole of the body would be considered sex to me; it would have to involve genital contact, however, I would class sado-masochism (SM) as sex regardless of whether there was contact or not. In these descriptions of lesbian sex, I have particularly highlighted those accounts which talk about the range of other behaviours, besides the genital, that the participant identifies as sexual. The point I am making is how all of these meanings can be accommodated in a single question which assumes we all share the same definition of – what the researchers had described as – the least ambiguous element of sexual identity. Moreover, in a study that recruits both heterosexuals and homosexuals, lesbian, gay and bisexual research participants are likely to assume that the concepts and meanings used relate to heterosexuality.

Concluding remarks about sampling

Probability methods can make a distinctive contribution to research among LGB communities because participants are selected randomly; they enable comparison with heterosexual participants who were recruited on the same basis; and they have considerable impact upon policy-making. But the description of random methods as an unproblematic 'gold-standard' of research (Solarz, 1999: 37) requires further analysis. Merely adding LGB people into population-based studies without systematic attention to these possible limitations may mean the replacement of one problem: lack of representativeness, with others: lack of attention to the ways in which heterosexism permeates the research process from the concepts used to sampling methods.

Developments in LGB non-probability research

The problems surrounding the recruitment of participants are not unique to LGB studies, but are common to all research among rare, hidden or sensitive populations. Examples of such populations include homeless people (Heckathorn, 2002) and IV drug users (Penrod et al., 2003; Thompson and Collins, 2002). Lee and Renzetti (1993) caution that sensitivity, rather than being attributable to the topic itself, is more to do with the relationship between the topic and the social context within which the research is conducted. These populations also lack a probability sampling frame – the homeless, for example, cannot be reached through household surveys or random digit-dialling (Heckathorn, 2002). Research on sensitive topics, then, has tended to have two contradictory outcomes: to inhibit adequate conceptualisation and measurement and has led to methodological advances in the form of technological innovation.

Location (or convenience) sampling

A popular method for sampling among LGB populations is through the use of locations known to be attended by large numbers of LGB people. In some respects, this method follows the pattern of early studies where researchers commonly recruited participants through gay bars. Annual Pride events – which take place in cities throughout the UK (and the rest of the world) – present an unparalleled opportunity for recruiting large numbers of LGB people. Sigma Research has been conducting studies of gay men's sexual behaviour for over a decade and obtains samples of approximately 5000 gay and bisexual men (e.g. Hickson et al., 2002). Pride events are no longer confined to major cities like Birmingham, Bristol and Glasgow, but smaller towns and cities not associated with large LGB populations – such as Bolton, Wakefield and Aberdeen – also hold regular Pride events. They thus enable researchers to achieve some geographical variability in their studies. Nor are Pride events limited to white, affluent LGBs who can afford high ticket prices: there are youth Prides in the UK, many events have retained their political origins and offer free entry, and Black Pride events are held in nine US cities (Battle et al., 2002). Moreover, location sampling facilitates the recruitment of hidden LGB groups; Keogh et al. recruited Black-Caribbean gay men through commercial gay venues with mainly black clientele and working class men through other targeted methods (2004a, 2004b). Location sampling, while offering a number of advantages over other methods, will only select LGB people who are sufficiently 'out' to be able to attend them. They may also be less likely to attract LGB people over the age of 60.

Snowball and chain-referral sampling

In snowball sampling, an initial sample of a target population is asked to identify other members of the population from within their personal networks, and they in turn are asked to identify others (Thompson and Collins, 2002). This method has been successful in recruiting adolescent smokers to studies. Rather than ask participants to put their peers at risk by disclosing their identity so that the researcher can make contact, many LGB researchers instead ask the referrer to pass on questionnaires directly. In this type of sampling, recruitment continues until all potential participants are contacted. Despite its name, snowball sampling does not lead to a growing mass of contacts, but rather a slow and uneven growth of additional points of contact. One of the limitations of the method is the tendency towards in-group recruitment: participants tend to recruit others who are like them. Ethnicity and gender affect who is sampled; Heckathorn (2002) found that white and Hispanic people, on the whole, recruit from within their own communities. The method also over-represents those with large personal networks because the number of potential recruitment paths leading to them is greater (Heckathorn, 2002).

Chain-referral is a sampling method which seeks to overcome some of these limitations by sampling among multiple social networks. It too relies on a series of participant referrals; however, a theoretical model is devised so multiple networks can be accessed. The chains of referral are carefully established at the outset by defining the population to be studied; decisions are made about the size of the sample so that statistical analysis can be conducted upon sub-samples (Penrod et al., 2003). Settings may be selected as potential sources of participants, for example, agencies that serve minority clientele; where possible, referrers are 'matched' on demographics with potential participants; participants may also be asked to distribute questionnaires only to peers who meet those people with socio-demographic characteristics who are most hidden. Heckathorn (2002) argues that chain-referral methods produce samples which have known levels of precision.

Telephone sampling

Telephone sampling has presented an interesting development in recent research among lesbians, gay men and bisexual people as it allows participants to retain their anonymity. It may be then a useful mechanism for encouraging participation from LGB people who are more likely to be closeted. Random digit-dialling (RDD) is the preferred method because the technique allows coverage of unlisted numbers (ex-directory) and anonymity – only the telephone number is known by the researcher. The method is expensive to operate, because it is unable to filter out business numbers and numbers which have not been allocated – typically resulting in a large number of irrelevant calls. Although telephone sampling using RDD is a probability sampling method, it has been adapted for use in LGB research. It has been used with some success to sample from communities in which lesbians and gay men are known to live in high concentrations, such as New York City and San Francisco. In these cities, the density of lesbian and gay residents is high enough to make initial household screening economically feasible. The benefits are that in highly populated areas they produce a sufficiently large sample of lesbians, gay men and bisexuals for analysis which is notably different from that produced through non-probability methods. By drawing a sample from a neighbourhood with a large population of lesbians, Meyer et al. (2002) expected to be able to make comparisons between heterosexual and lesbian/bisexual women with the assumption that they would be similar in demographic characteristics and health outcomes. While the two groups did not differ in regard to 'race' or physical health, the lesbian and bisexual women were younger, more educated, more likely to be unemployed and had significantly worse mental health scores. In accounting for the particularly high prevalence of lesbians in the sample – 14 per cent identified as lesbian – in comparison to 1.8 per cent in an RDD survey conducted nationally (Bradford et al., 1997) – the researchers note that the neighbourhood was selected because of the known high density of lesbians living there and this may have facilitated self-disclosure. Even though the neighbourhood was known to have a high density of lesbians and one would assume a more permissive environment, 2.5 per cent did not disclose their sexual identity.

Contrary to expectations, telephone sampling can also introduce 'selection bias' (Solarz, 1999: 121). While those lesbians and gay men who reside in high-density lesbian and gay neighbourhoods may have similar demographic characteristics to the heterosexuals in the sample, they may differ from lesbians and gay men in the population as a whole. High-density lesbian, gay and bisexual neighbourhoods are usually located in large urban centres where rents may often be high: the technique may reproduce some of the limitations associated with non-probability sampling by over-recruiting those from higher socio-economic groups. This in turn may have an impact on the findings; in Meyer et al.'s study (2002), relatively high numbers of lesbians were 'out' to family, co-workers and health care providers and high levels of disclosure are usually associated with good mental health. Despite this, the mental health of lesbians and bisexual women was poorer than that of the heterosexual women in the study; the findings may suggest that lesbians with less social support and living in more conservative communities may experience even worse levels of mental health than those reported in the study. However, lifestyle changes in relation to telephone usage may undermine these efforts. In a general discussion of telephone surveys, Collins (2002) points to a number of potentially serious future problems including the trend towards using mobile phones as the main means of connection and communication, answerphone machines used as barriers to unwanted calls, lines that connect to fax machines but also cover a residential line and, a problem particular to the UK context, where subscriber numbers conceal digits that represent exchange codes.

Other methods of recruiting LGB to studies

Researchers among LGB populations have made innovations to existing methods with purposive samples drawn from among recipients of health services (Bailey et al., 2000; Gruskin et al., 2001); lesbian and gay community events or venues (Henderson et al., 2002; Hickson et al., 1998; Nardone et al., 2001); lesbian and gay social, political or sporting organisations (Bhugra, 1997; Galop, 2001); lesbian and gay publications (Diamant et al., 2000); mailing lists and conferences; the use of non-LGB sources such as bookshops and trade unions (Morris and Rothblum, 1999); and public sector organisations, such as local NHS trusts, which are known to employ relatively large numbers of LGB (Sexuality Matters, 2005). The internet may improve the accessibility of research; researchers design a web-based questionnaire and use LGB internet sites to recruit research participants.

Multiple sampling frames

By combining sampling methods, researchers hope to obtain a more diverse sample than is possible through the use of a single sampling strategy. In the Lesbians and Health Care Survey, a range of sampling strategies was used to increase the diversity of the achieved sample (Fish, 1999). The study was conducted over a 12-month period and publicised through local, regional and national LGB publications; a wide range of groups were contacted up and down the country including lesbian and gay switchboards, women's centres and health groups, lesbian organisations for particular groups including disabled, older, younger, black, and bisexual lesbians – and these groups were particularly identified in recruitment letters. Participants were recruited through snowballing sampling, six Pride or similar events, alternative bookshops, a lesbian health newsletter, trade unions, university LGB societies, lesbian sexual health clinics, social groups and cancer organisations (the study topic concerned breast and cervical cancer screening); in addition, personal contact was found to encourage participation and a number of venues were visited as well as gay bars. In all, 486 letters were sent and more than 200 phone calls were made. Because geographic distribution was important for a national survey, a matrix was devised to ensure participation from each of the 122 postcode areas throughout the UK. Where there were no or few returns, efforts were made to contact lesbians living in those areas. The final sample included participation from lesbians living from Cornwall to the Outer Hebrides and living in all but five of the postcode areas.

Assessing the impact of source of recruitment on the sample achieved

Recent research has been conducted to assess the effectiveness of different methods in obtaining participants both in terms of numbers and diversity. One of the first studies to assess whether the source of recruitment resulted in differences in the sample composition was Martin and Dean's (1993) study where they found that the population of gay men recruited through a public health clinic was quite different to that obtained through other sources – they were younger, had lower annual incomes, were primarily African-American or Hispanic and less likely to be a member of a gay group or organisation.

Rothblum et al. (2002) used different methods to sample participants and found that over 30 per cent of their sample was recruited through local or state periodicals, while national periodicals were the most effective means of recruiting black lesbians and those with less education. The ESTHER study of health risks in lesbians found that mailing lists (49 per cent) was the most effective of the strategies used, with community events (21 per cent), organisations (15 per cent), and personal networks (15 per cent) achieving varying degrees of success (Rothblum et al., 2002). In the latter study, strategies that were more successful at recruiting black lesbians included recruitment through community events – rather than organisations even though some of the targeted organisations included African-American women – while the use of organisations appeared to be a better recruiting strategy for older lesbians (Rothblum et al., 2002).

The use of control groups

Researchers have recently looked to other ways of ensuring the rigour and validity of the studies they seek to undertake. One innovation has been to use lesbians and their heterosexual sisters as a control group (Rothblum and Factor, 2001). Although the study was conducted using non-probability methods – participants were recruited through the US Gayellow pages – both groups were recruited through the same method and thus a comparable demographic control group was ensured. The method controlled for 'race', age, parental socio-economic status and parental education.

Conclusion

Because probability methods form the sampling paradigm in research, reviewers for high quality peer-reviewed journals insist on their use. Lesbian, gay and bisexual researchers often fail to get their work published because they have used non-probability methods. This criterion does not appear to be applied in quite the same way to similar health and social care research among (presumed) heterosexual hard-to-reach populations, such as drug-users or homeless people, because it is immediately apparent that traditional methods of contacting them are not relevant. It would appear, then, that LGB researchers must provide additional evidence of rigour. There seem to be a number of reasons for this cautionary approach. It is partly because the socio-demographic characteristics of the heterosexual population are already known and so the homeless (for example) are readily acknowledged as a sub-population. It may be partly because the LGB population is deemed too small to be worthy of research. But it also seems that LGB research is considered to be inevitably biased and its use of non-probability methods is seen as an indication of this. Finally, reviewers believe that LGB health and social care needs are the same as those of heterosexuals and therefore research is not needed. These issues illustrate the need for a comprehensive examination of the ways in which heterosexism permeates the process of research.

5
What are the Demographic Characteristics of the LGB Population?

How many LGB people are there in the UK?

Numbers are invested with considerable importance in western culture. Not only do we have a fascination for those things that can be counted, but numbers offer tangible reassurance about what is known. For LGB populations, numbers hold particular power because judgements about the relative size of the population have often been made to support or deny claims to the community's significance. In the early 1950s, Kinsey and his colleagues (1948, 1953) shocked the US with findings that same-sex sexual behaviour was much more prevalent than had previously been thought (the books were also widely read in the UK). Kinsey et al.'s research was used (by others) to produce one of the most enduring 'facts' about LGB people: the statistic that they formed 1 in 10 of the population. The statistic had currency for almost two decades, but by the early 1990s, two large-scale studies had downgraded the LGB population to 1 in 50 (Wellings et al., 1994; Laumann et al., 1994). Both teams of researchers argued that their findings challenged previous calculations; in particular, Laumann et al. (1994) sought to debunk the 10 per cent myth. Their esti-mates of 3.6 per cent for men and 1.8 per cent for women shaped beliefs about the size of the population for the following decade. Some LGB researchers reacted angrily to these calculations: one argued that the sample of lesbians achieved in Wellings et al. (1994) was smaller than her own circle of friends and acquaintances (Stanley, 1995).

Why is this preoccupation with statistics so important in LGB research? Statistics have political significance. Estimates of small numbers have been used, especially by the Christian right wing in the US, to dismiss LGB civil rights claims as a waste of taxpayers' money (Young and Meyer, 2005); the continuing invisibility of LGB populations is an outcome of heterosexism. Larger estimates offer the potential that LGB concerns will be recognised and addressed. However, the relative size of LGB populations is no guarantee for social policy initiatives. The LGB population in Brighton and Hove is the city's largest minority. Yet, despite a comprehensive health and social care needs strategy, no public body has been charged with its implementation.

Available statistics about LGB people

Statistics about lesbians and gay men should be approached with caution. Census data, believed to offer the most reliable information about national populations, have provided even lower estimates than random surveys. The US census estimates the proportion of LGB same-sex couples at just over 1 per cent of the US population, while the UK census provides the lower estimate of 0.19 per cent (of the 40 666 546 couples in England and Wales, only 78 522 were same-sex couples). There are three explanations for this under-reporting.

First, demographers in the US suggest that only about one-third of LGB couples report themselves as such in the census (Black et al., 2000): that is, LGB people intentionally refuse to self-report. The census differs in important ways from other surveys; although census data are confidential for 100 years, they are not anonymous. Some respondents may be reluctant to provide confirmation in writing of their sexual identity. There is further evidence supporting this explanation: when the national survey (Johnson et al., 2001) introduced anonymous reporting of sexual identity, it found that the numbers of women reporting same-sex relationships had increased threefold in a ten-year period and gay men formed over 10 per cent of the population of Greater London. The 2000 US census reported similar increases over the previous decade.

Second, none of the large population-based studies – the census, the General Household Survey (GHS) or the Labour Force Survey (LFS) – directly asks participants about their sexual identity. Instead, in the census, these data are imputed. In the GHS, questions are asked about household size, marital status and cohabitation, while in the LFS, participants are invited to respond to an item – 'unmarried partner' – in order to identify their same-sex relationship. Current legislation in the UK (notwithstanding the recent introduction of Civil Partnerships) does not entitle same-sex couples to marry; some may then believe that the item applies only to heterosexual couples. Moreover, although census researchers recognise that the challenge is to 'count everyone in' in their list of under-enumerated groups who require special arrangements to be included, LGB people are not identified (ONS, 2001).

Third, while the census samples only same-sex couples in order to enable comparison with heterosexual couples, this may also contribute to under-reporting. Among LGB communities there has been a consistent finding, in the US, UK and Sweden, that LGB people are more likely to live alone. There are fluctuating estimations, however, of the rates at which they do so. Some US studies suggest that as many as 72 per cent of gay men and 56 per cent of lesbians live alone. UK studies suggest smaller differences: 17 per cent of LGB in comparison to 12 per cent of heterosexuals live alone. Data based on people living in couple relationships may not provide reliable estimates of LGB people in the UK. There are thus concerns about the ability of the census to provide accurate calculations about the size of the LGB population (Black et al., 2000). Furthermore, US demographers suggest that there is inconsistency within the census: the LGB population estimates vary for California by 13 per cent; while those for North Dakota vary by as much as 220 per cent (www.gaydemographics.org, retrieved 10 October 2005).

Notwithstanding these provisos, the UK Census – which collected data about same-sex couples for the first time in 2001 – provides important first information about the LGB population. Although only 81 298 people reported that they were living as a same-sex couple, the data provide detailed information about where they lived (at ward level) in England, Wales, Scotland and Northern Ireland.

Where do LGB people live?

Most importantly, the notion of a community completely concentrated in urban environments is debunked by UK census data. Contrary to popular misconceptions, there are no vast swathes of so-called 'middle England' uninhabited by lesbians, gay men and bisexuals. The UK comedy programme *Little Britain* satirised this in the sketch 'the only gay in the village', but the census shows that even in the remote corner of north west Scotland, 14 people on the Shetland Islands identified themselves as living in same-sex couples (www.gaydemographics.org/UK/local.html, retrieved 10 October 2005). LGB have been shown to live in almost all of the 438 Local Authority areas in the UK (in only two places in Northern Ireland did same-sex couples not identify themselves in the census). Table 5.1 lists the six UK cities with more than 1000 LGB residents ranked in order of the highest number.

It possibly comes as no surprise that Brighton and Hove is the UK's fastest growing LGB community; over the past decade many LGB people have relocated from other parts of the country to the medium-sized

Table 5.1 Highest concentrations of LGB people in UK cities (outside London)

Local authority	Number of same-sex couples	Proportion of total population (%)
Brighton & Hove	2554	2.49
Glasgow	1594	0.80
Edinburgh	1442	0.76
Birmingham	1348	0.35
Manchester	1290	1.03
Leeds	1230	0.38

(Data derived from www.gaydemographics.com)

Table 5.2 Highest concentrations of LGB people in key inner London boroughs

London	Number of same-sex couples	Proportion of total population (%)
Lambeth	1716	2.07
Southwark	1230	1.54
Islington	1180	2.15
Wandsworth	1134	1.20
Lewisham	1070	1.17
Camden	1046	1.69
Hackney	1028	1.68
Tower Hamlets	1004	1.56

(Data derived from www.gaydemographics.com)

coastal town. But it is surprising that Manchester – widely thought of as the gay capital of the north – should have approximately half of Brighton's LGB population and that it is only marginally larger than that of Leeds. The two major cities in Scotland each had more than 1000 LGB same-sex couples, while the two remaining capital cities of the UK – Cardiff and Belfast – both had relatively small numbers of people reporting. Other cities, where large numbers might be expected, such as Nottingham, Bristol and Newcastle, had less than 1000 LGB reporting.

The inner boroughs of London are reputed to have large LGB populations. Table 5.2 gives the numbers and proportions for the most densely populated London boroughs. Although these figures are low in comparison to NATSAL 2000 where 5.5 per cent of men had a same-sex relationship in the past five years, they are interesting in so far as Camden, Islington and Hackney would probably be seen as the Inner London boroughs with the highest numbers of LGB. In fact, the top two positions are occupied by boroughs not usually associated with high populations of LGB. In comparison to the rest of the UK population, their size and proportion are larger, but the figures are much smaller than those provided by NATSAL 2000.

In the neighbourhood statistics, the census reveals that of the 75 744 LGB people living in England, 46 per cent of them live in London and the south east. There seem to be two possible explanations for these findings. On the one hand, they may indicate that while LGB are geographically distributed throughout the UK, they are more likely than heterosexuals to live in urban environments. On the other, it may be that LGB who live in wealthier areas, have higher social status, and, with the relative anonymity provided by large cities, may be more likely to disclose their sexual identity. The UK census findings which indicate a high concentration of LGB in the south east and London may have implications for our understanding of LGB incomes. If studies are more likely to recruit samples from the south east and London – areas known for higher average annual incomes – then data about LGB affluence may be an outcome of sampling bias.

There may also be differences between lesbians and gay men in terms of their geographic distribution. In a comparison between two UK community-based samples, one of gay men (Hickson et al., 1998) and the other of lesbians (Fish, 2002), gay men were more likely than lesbians to live in London and the south east: 50 per cent of gay men lived in these regions in comparison to 40 per cent of lesbians.

High concentrations of LGB seem to be a more likely characteristic of the US population than they are of the UK. There are several US counties with a nil return for same-sex couples. Moreover, US research suggests that lesbians and gay men are concentrated in twenty cities: a gay man is 12 times more likely to live in San Francisco than his heterosexual counterpart. In addition, in comparison to their heterosexual sisters, lesbians have been found to be more geographically mobile and to live further away from their parents.

Unlike the US census, which provides a wealth of information about home ownership, education, employment, occupation, children, disability and years living together, the UK census only provides data about geographic location for LGB people. For this reason, the following sections draw upon a range of sources in their discussion.

What is known about the social characteristics of LGB people?

Income

While the size of the LGB population has been a matter of considerable concern, there is also a persistent and pervasive stereotype that LGB people are more likely to be in the ABC1 social bracket and have higher than average incomes. The perception of affluence has also been fostered by some within LGB communities. Gay businesses, seeking to attract mainstream advertising revenues, have commissioned market research which has shown high disposable incomes among LGBs. The myth of the so-called *Pink Pound* has been derived, not from population-based surveys, but through the readership of glossy magazines, such as *Gay Times* and *Diva*. However, the target audience of any glossy magazine is not typical of average adults. African-American readers of *Ebony*, *Essence* and *Jet* magazines earned up to 80 per cent more than the average African-American (Badgett, 1998). Market research showing the high earning power of the readership of *Gay Times* is perfectly legitimate; the use of such research to make generalisations about the relative wealth of the LGB population in the UK is not. Perceptions about LGB affluence may have unforeseen consequences: data have been used in court actions in the US to dismiss their claims for civil rights (Plumb, 2001). Lesbians and gay men are believed, by some, to comprise an economic elite who have disproportionate political power and are insulated from discrimination because of their affluent status. The *Pink Pound* made (certain groups of) LGB highly visible within the economy, but the price of that visibility has been to create a stereotype of wealth and privilege. Efforts have also been made to counter heterosexist assumptions that LGB were employed in only a limited range of occupations at the margins of society. LGB were shown to be employed in a range of professional occupations and were thus both capable and trustworthy. But these arguments have also been taken, by opponents to LGB civil rights, as indications of their relative privilege.

White gay men form the segment of the LGB population most associated with affluence. In stark contrast, analyses of government population-based surveys seem to indicate that the average gay man earns up to 5 per cent less than the average heterosexual man, although there was no difference between men who lived in London (Arabsheibani et al., 2004). In the UK, the earnings differential appears to favour lesbians: they have been found to earn up to 11 per cent more than comparable heterosexual women (Arabsheibani et al., 2004). The UK results are surprising in the light of long-standing evidence which indicates a gender pay gap: among heterosexuals, men are likely to earn more than women.

US studies have also analysed income (Black et al., 2000). Among women, the findings are contradictory. Analysis of different studies in the US has shown the full spectrum of relative earnings: lesbians earn less, the same and more than the average heterosexual woman (Badgett, 1998). Moreover, the apparent income advantage disappears once the longer hours and more weeks of the year that lesbians work are taken into account. Wage differentials are highly segmented by 'race'. Black female same-sex couples in the US earn approximately $9000 less than their black heterosexual counterparts and $18 000 less than their white same-sex counterparts. Black male same-sex couples earn $2000 less than their black heterosexual counterparts and $20 000 less than white same-sex counterparts (Dang and Frazer, 2005). A number of other factors contribute to the likelihood of higher earning potential and as indicators of social class including education, occupation, employment status, home ownership and family structure. Three further demographic factors are considered – 'race' and ethnicity, service in the armed forces and collective living and working arrangements – which provide important data about the characteristics of LGB populations.

Education

Among US gay men, almost 24 per cent have college degrees; the corresponding rate for married men is 17 per cent (Black et al., 2000). To test the reliability of their findings, the researchers found that the distribution of education among gay men's fathers was almost identical to that of the heterosexual men in their analyses and they argue that the data provide tentative evidence that gay men have higher levels of educational attainment. When Badgett (1998) controlled for education, location, race, age, disability and number of children, gay men earned 27 per cent less than comparable heterosexual men in the US. Badgett (1998) theorised that the findings for gay men suggest workplace discrimination. Similar levels of educational qualifications have been found among US lesbians, of whom 25 per cent have a college education in comparison to 16 per cent of married women. Research which used heterosexual sisters as a control group found that US lesbians had significantly higher levels of education, no difference in occupational levels and no difference in individual or household income (Rothblum and Factor, 2001). Other studies have also suggested that lesbians have higher educational qualifications than heterosexual women; typically, higher levels of educational achievement correlate with higher income (and consequently social class), but this is not the case for lesbians surveyed in the US.

In their meta-analyses, Arabsheibani et al. (2004) found that around 36 per cent of LGB (among lesbians this was slightly more) have a degree or above compared to 15 per cent of their heterosexual counterparts. Some UK community-based surveys have also suggested that lesbians and gay men are more highly educated than the population as a whole (Fish, 2002; Hickson et al., 1998). In the Lesbians and Health Care Survey (LHCS), the sample was much more highly educated: only 39 per cent had *not* received a higher education in comparison with 86 per cent of all women in the UK. Of interest is an early British study (Kenyon, 1968) which included a control group of heterosexual women; it lends support to findings that lesbians may be more highly educated than heterosexual women. The study found that more lesbians went to university (and more left school at 15 without any qualifications). Among gay men, 25 per cent of men had no qualifications or only GSCEs or equivalent and were more highly educated than the adult male population. Hickson et al. (1998) argue that this is the case for all samples of homosexually active men recruited from all gay settings. Education is important to experiences of health care because it is said to help people become articulate health care consumers.

Occupation

Demographers have analysed US data about occupation. Of the 476 occupations listed in the US census, 15 occupations accounted for 25 per cent of LGB people. Those occupations which tended to be favoured by gay men included designers, car mechanics, drivers and truckers, janitors and general managers. The most common occupations for lesbians included child care workers, counsellors, accountants, waitresses and solicitors.

In the UK, 44 per cent of gay men and 37 per cent of lesbians are in the professional, managerial and intermediate registrar general classifications compared to 35 per cent and 21 per cent of male and female heterosexuals (Arabsheibani et al., 2004). Lesbians and gay men were more likely to work in social and community work sectors and in larger firms. In the LHCS, occupations among lesbians included nurses and a range of other health professionals, teachers, lecturers, social workers, police officers, engineers as well as library assistants, drivers and factory workers. These 1049 responses were coded according to the census, which outlines the job titles for over 370 different occupations where they are grouped with up to nine other similar jobs. Each of these is categorised into ten broad occupational groups (which are then accorded a social class). Using baseline data from the census, there are the same proportions of managers and administrators in the LHCS sample as there are in the female population in general (11 per cent). However, the percentages of LHCS participants who are employed in professional occupations is almost three times greater (29 per cent vs. 10 per cent) than in the female population (Matheson and Summerfield, 2000). For those in 'associate professional' occupations the differential is more than three times greater (35 per cent vs. 11 per cent). Conversely, there are fewer lesbians in the LHCS employed in those occupations 'lower down' the scale, than in the general population: for example, there is less than one-quarter of the proportionate numbers in clerical and secretarial positions (6.3 per cent vs. 26 per cent). Overall, the proportion of lesbians in the study who occupy professional and associate professional occupations is considerably higher than in the female population as a whole.

Employment status

Less attention appears to have been paid to women located at the other end of the employment spectrum. The LHCS found similar proportions of lesbians were economically inactive to the UK female population (27 per cent vs. 28 per cent); of particular note are lesbians who are unemployed. UK national data (Matheson and Summerfield, 2000) suggest that 3.5 per cent of the female population were unemployed; the LHCS found almost three times that number were unemployed (9.5 per cent). These data suggest that lesbians may be clustered at both the higher and lower ends of income scales. Furthermore, a survey in Brighton, a city particularly associated with upwardly mobile LGB found higher levels of unemployment: despite the fact that LGB were more likely to hold degrees, 31 per cent were unemployed.

Family structure

The family structure of LGB relationships has often been cited as the reason for their higher incomes: they are believed to be less likely to have interrupted their careers in order to care for children and being childfree means they have higher disposable incomes. Analyses of two combined US studies suggest that a substantial number of same-sex couples currently live with children: about 28 per cent of lesbians and 14 per cent of gay men (Black et al., 2000). However, heterosexual women were more likely than their lesbian sisters to be living with children (Rothblum and Factor, 2001). In black female same-sex households, children are raised at twice the rate reported by white same-sex couples (61 per cent vs. 38 per cent)

(Dang and Frazer, 2005). There may be an increased likelihood of kinship care among black families, where same-sex couples may raise a niece, nephew or grandchild (Battle et al., 2000).

Home ownership

Finally, home ownership is also an indicator of relative wealth. In the analysis of the US census, the rate of home ownership was lower for part-nered gay and lesbians' households than for married couple households. If they did own a house, same-sex couples were likely to have more expen-sive homes than their heterosexual counterparts. Only 50 per cent of black same-sex couples are less likely to report home ownership than are black heterosexual couples (Dang and Frazer, 2005). Sexuality Matters (2005) found that LGB people were twice as likely as heterosexuals living in an East Midlands city to live in privately rented accommodation.

'Race' and ethnicity

The 2000 US census recorded 600 000 same sex-couples, of whom 85 000 were black; this figure represents 14 per cent of all same-sex people living in coupled relationships (Dang and Frazer, 2005). Non-probability studies have been conducted among black LGB communities – one of the largest was undertaken at nine different Pride events in the US (Battle et al., 2000). The characteristics of this sample of 2645 black LGB people showed that they were more highly educated and earned slightly more household income than the general black population. Those surveyed were more likely to work in a professional job and less likely to work in the service sec-tor. Nearly one-quarter worked for the government while three-quarters worked in the private sector.

In the UK, there is little information about the characteristics of black LGB populations. Although participants in the LHCS were predominantly of white ethnic origin, the numbers of black lesbians (Black-African, Black-Caribbean, Black-Other) who took part in the survey were twice their proportions in the population as a whole at the time the survey was conducted. Comparisons are made in Table 5.3 to the UK population.

Although a slightly smaller proportion in the LHCS described themselves as belonging to one of the 'non-white' categories than in the LFS or OPCS samples, there are important differences in the way in which the data are analysed in these three data sets. In both the Labour Force Survey and the census (OPCS, 1995), the ethnic minority totals of these samples included respondents who had described themselves as belonging to the category 'other groups'. The researchers, during analysis of the data, reallocated those respondents from 'other groups' to the survey's ethnic

Table 5.3   Comparisons of ethnic origin between LHCS and other UK data

Ethnic group	Lesbians and Health Care Survey (%)	Labour Force Survey (%)	Proportion of population in UK 1991 OPCS (%)
White	90	94.2	94.5
Black*(-African)	0.5	}1.1	} 1.6
Black-Caribbean	2.1	}	}
Black-Other	0.9	}	}
Indian	0.1	1.4	1.5
Pakistani	0.1	0.9	0.9
Bangladeshi		0.2	0.3
Chinese	0.1	0.3	0.3
Asian-Other	0.6		
Other groups	4	1.0	0.9
Not stated	1	0.9	n/a
More than one box ticked	0.3		
Totals	99.6	100	100

OPCS 1995
*includes 'Black-Caribbean', 'Black-African', 'Black-Other', in OPCS and LFS data

minority categories. (Without this subsequent recategorisation by the researchers, these 'other' categories would be reduced to 3.9 per cent in the LFS and 4.6 per cent in the census). In the LHCS the additional 4 per cent of participants who described their ethnic origin as 'Other' were *not* reallocated in this way (if they were, the total proportion of participants from ethnic minorities would be 8.4 per cent). A further important difference between the census and other large data sets is that the census is a compulsory survey with legal penalties for refusal which means that refusal rates are low (OPCS, 1995: 121). In addition, there were no 'no responses' to the question about ethnic origin in the census data, because not stated answers are imputed (OPCS, 1995: 122). It was neither possible (nor ethically desirable) to reallocate the 1 per cent of 'no responses' in the LHCS to the existing ethnic origin categories.

A significant omission in the LHCS is the non-participation of lesbians from Bangladeshi communities. In comparison, Hickson et al.'s National Gay Men's Sex Survey (NGMSS) (1998), which has a sample that is four times larger than the LHCS – and therefore one would expect a larger sample to include at least a small number of 'hard-to-access' groups – found that fewer than five men indicated that their ethnicity was Bangladeshi. This may suggest that participation needs to be more actively encouraged from amongst the Bangladeshi population.

Service in the armed forces

The US census suggests that gay men are much less likely than heterosexual men to be veterans and lesbians are much more likely to have served in the military (Black et al., 2000). Black lesbians are nearly four times as likely as their heterosexual counterparts to report veteran status and they are discharged from the military at rates far exceeding their representation under the *Don't Ask, Don't Tell* policy (Dang and Frazer, 2005).

Collective living and working arrangements

One factor, not previously discussed in US demographic studies among lesbians, is the social phenomenon of collective living and working arrangements which were a particular feature of lesbian separatism. Such arrangements may affect where lesbians live and how much they earn. It is not clear whether such communes were long since abandoned in the US (Faderman, 1992), but in the UK there are signs of their continued existence. In the 1980s, a number of UK lesbians chose to migrate to smaller communities in the north where living and housing costs were cheaper. This migration seems to be reflected in recent analyses of UK census data which show that the highest number of lesbians per head in the UK live in the small market town of Hebden Bridge, in North Yorkshire.

Todmodern, in nearby Lancashire, is known anecdotally as another lesbian enclave; there are also reports of small, thriving lesbian communities living in Gwynedd in North Wales, the Isle of Mull and the Outer Hebrides in Scotland. Such communities owe their existence to lesbian feminist critiques of institutionalised heterosexism and gender roles. While the current challenge to traditional ways of living and working are no longer so widespread or so evident, a minority of lesbians appear to integrate this politicised commitment into their lives in a number of ways. My theory is based on the observation of three phenomena: first, that some lesbians leave professional (or other) occupations and take up non-traditional jobs in their communities such as painting and decorating or plumbing; second, some lesbians reduce their hours to part-time working in order to fund an activity into which they put their energies: for example, in order to support creative ventures or political activity; third, some lesbians appear to reject workplace hierarchies and instead of moving up the career ladder, they choose to move sideways. Some lesbians with political perspectives (and other groups also) continue the self-sufficiency movements of the late 1970s: they grow their own organic vegetables, take holidays in the UK and make efforts to reduce their consumption of the world's resources. Consequently, they have reduced their need for high wages. This is not to say that other groups may not similarly abandon the 'rat race', but that lesbians may be more likely to be in a position to do this, because they may be less likely to have dependent children. My argument is not that these phenomena are unique to lesbians, but that they engage in collective living and working arrangements in greater proportions than either gay men or heterosexuals. I am not aware of a similar social phenomenon among gay men; however, in the 1980s a housing co-op, Wild Lavender, was set up in Leeds by gay men who wished to live co-operatively.

Conclusion

Existing sources of information are likely to provide only partial data about LGB populations. There are a number of reasons, discussed in this and the previous chapter, why LGB may refuse, or fail, to identify themselves in the census and other population-based surveys. However, the proportions of LGB who disclosed their sexual identity increased almost threefold when researchers introduced anonymous reporting in a national survey (Johnson et al., 2001). Such random population-based studies usually employ face-to-face interview as a means of gathering data. By contrast, community-based surveys are likely to over-recruit educated LGB because they typically use self-completion questionnaires which are more likely to include those with good literacy skills. Nevertheless, data are emerging for the first time about the nature of LGB populations around the world: Uruguay, Spain, Australia, New Zealand and Canada have introduced questions in their national censuses, while other countries, notably Norway and Holland, have begun to collect data about same-sex domestic partnership registrations or marriages. They may enable international comparisons and provide data about LGB population trends. Following the implementation of the Civil Partnerships legislation, the government has, for the first time, provided an estimate of 6 per cent of the total population, which means that there are about 3.6 million lesbian, gay and bisexual people in the UK.

Part II
Exemplars of Heterosexism from Research

6
Disclosure and Non-disclosure: Lesbians' Strategies of Accommodation and Resistance in their Interactions with Health Professionals

Concepts of the closet and coming out

Coming out refers to two phenomenological experiences: acknowledging one's identity to oneself and telling others that one is lesbian, gay or bisexual. Although coming out begins when individuals define themselves, the acceptance of a 'homosexual' identity is characterised by disclosing it to others. There is a well-established body of work in relation to the first experience, but disclosure to others has only recently been a topic for investigation.

The necessity of coming out is linked to notions of the closet. The closet has often been described as a space where LGB identities can be kept separate and hidden. In some depictions, the closet is a prison in which the gay person is kept captive; in others, the closet is a geography, most frequently an underworld characterised by bars and clubs, which are distinct from the world of the heterosexual mainstream. Its secretive character offers protection from unwanted exposure. In archetypal narratives of the closet, the individual maintains a public and socially approved persona as heterosexual that is separate from their private gay identity. Because those who inhabit the closet fear discovery, they have usually told no one (or very few people), typically because they feel shame or guilt (Seidman et al., 1999). Recently, the closet has come to characterise certain individuals. Such notions have led researchers to investigate the demographic characteristics associated with being out. Harry (1993) proposed that people in artistic occupations and some service industries were most likely to be out, while those in traditional professions, such as teachers, doctors, and those working in science and technology were least likely to be out. Those with the highest and low-est income levels were also most likely to be out. Other researchers have suggested that certain personality types are most likely to be closeted. They are people who lead sad and false lives: the socially isolated, older people, those who have only recently acknowledged an LGB identity and those who are religious. In whatever way the closet is depicted, it remains the defining feature of LGB oppression (Kosofsky-Sedgwick, 1993).

Coming out is a momentous act in the lives of lesbians and gay men. It is often described as a once-in-a-lifetime event – a 'road to Damascus' experience (Davies, 1992: 75) – in which the newly acknowledged LGB person flings open the closet door and announces to the world: I am a gay man/lesbian. When Ellen DeGeneres came out, it was a single event in which her identity was acknowledged to the world (although there had been many hints and clues along the way). Coming out was not merely an individual act of self-affirmation, but also a key strategy in building a movement. The 1969 Stonewall rebellion collectivised LGB identities and the slogan 'out of the closets and onto the streets' encap-sulated this sense of public identities. Lesbians and gay men proclaimed their identities 'from the housetops' (Gross, 1993: 146) and being out was a political position which would inevitably lead to the end of anti-gay oppression and the achievement of civil rights.

In contrast to these accounts which represent coming out as a single, irrevocable event, in other narratives, coming out is described as a process by which one's gay identity becomes increasingly public and is openly expressed to everyone. Disclosure is incremental and unidirectional: it first occurs with a trusted member of one's intimate circle, usually a friend or a sibling; then to family and acquaintances, co-workers and the public at large – like ripples on a pond to ever 'widening circles of people' (Gerstel et al., 1989: 87). These narratives characterise a highly dichotomised phenomenon in which a person moves from total secrecy to total open-ness. The closet evokes tangibility and permanence: it is monolithic and static. Its opposite – coming out – is conceived of as a single event or a steady progress towards greater openness. These discursive strategies have shaped conceptions about what it means to be in the closet and what it means to be out. The concepts refer to opposite states of being and are predicated upon beliefs about separate spaces and double lives.

Instead of a separate, passive space, Kosofsky-Sedgwick proposes that the closet encroaches on everyday life: 'the deadly elasticity of hetero-sexist presumption means that . . . people find new walls springing up around them' (1993: 46). Because heterosexuality is all-pervasive, even the most openly gay people continually deal with decisions about disclosure or concealment. Every encounter with a new employer or work colleague, new friends or acquaintances, a new doctor or social worker, solicitor or teacher, neighbour or landlord/landlady presents LGB people with decisions about concealment or disclosure. The closet is actively constructed by the regime of compulsory heterosexuality: people are presumed to be heterosexual unless they declare themselves otherwise. This conceptual understanding of the closet allows for new analyses which, rather than polarising disclosure and non-disclosure, instead show them to be strategies which are situation-contingent.

Is the concept of the closet still relevant?

Some contend that the closet is no longer relevant in the lives of lesbians and gay men (Seidman et al., 1999). The contemporary landscape of social inclusion and diversity is steadily moving towards granting LGB people the same rights as those enjoyed by heterosexuals. Because of the new climate of openness, they argue, there is no longer any need for LGB people to be closeted. The social milieu has never been more favourable for coming out. The British Social Attitudes Survey reveals that people in Britain are now more 'tolerant' of homosexuality than ever before. Lesbians (who have always occupied a less visible position than gay men) are seen to inhabit all aspects of public life; there is an out lesbian MP (Angela Eagle), a lesbian Tory candidate for selection (Margot James) and *Diva*, the UK lesbian life and style magazine, featured an article about 100 high-profile lesbians working in sport, politics, business, the arts, academia and the media. Not so long ago, there were few representations of lesbians in television except as objects of derision or pity: now politicians and others in public life speak out in support of lesbian and gay equality. Being a lesbian or a gay man is no longer an impediment to success, a matter for subterfuge or potential for blackmail, and lesbians and gay men will no longer be hounded from public office because their identity has become known. Coming out is overwhelmingly considered to be the norm and the term itself has entered the everyday lexicon of the mainstream. Coming out of the closet has become a popular metaphor for the disclosure of *any* secret. People have come out as asexual, fashion designers and big women, but it is not only people who can exit the closet; India came out to declare its nuclear weapons capacity. In these instances, it describes *any* public utterance about something which is denigrated that one wants to take pride in (or announce to the world). The effect of this seems to render coming out inconsequential and commonplace.

Yet if such social transformations had taken place, and the closet had all but disappeared, one would expect this to be reflected in public life. In 2001, the UK census collected details for the first time about the numbers of LGB people living in same-sex relationships. Because the census records information about every household in the UK (people face fines if they do not complete it), it is said to provide a unique snapshot about contemporary social life. One would expect – if disclosure was no longer an issue – that it would provide accurate information about the LGB population. Information from the census indicates that there are 81 298 same-sex couples living in the UK. Recent government estimates suggest that the UK LGB population is 3.6 million. There appear to be two possible explanations for this discrepancy: either there are very few LGB people in the UK; or relatively few LGB people are prepared to disclose their sexual identity in a census which records their name and address (even though this information is not publicly available).

These discontinuities may also be accounted for in the different ways being out is managed in the lives of LGB people. Seidman et al. (1999) contend that many people have integrated their sexual identity in their personal lives, but in institutional settings they are less likely to routinely disclose. Even though many lesbians and gay men are out to family and friends, this does not always seem to be a simple matter. While many lesbians had come out to one or more family members, they described situations where the information had been passed on by a third party, some had had the information forced out of them, and others had come out to stop gossip (Markowe, 1996). Coming out in institutional settings may present further challenges. In health care, the self – the body, behaviour and personal life – is subject to (sometimes intense) scrutiny when any user of health care is at their most vulnerable. It is in this curious mix of the intensely personal in an institutional setting where an analysis of the ways in which lesbians, gay men and bisexuals negotiate disclosure and non-disclosure is particularly productive.

Disclosure and non-disclosure in health care

Coming out to a health care worker has been a common theme in lesbian health research and, more recently, in the health of gay men (Keogh et al., 2004b). Of particular concern have been such questions as: How many lesbians and gay men have disclosed to their health care provider? Is disclosure facilitated by the attitudes of staff? Are those who disclose more likely to be out to family and friends? (Martinson et al.,

1996). Less consideration has been devoted to the ways in which disclosure and non-disclosure are accomplished in health care settings.

Reasons for disclosure and non-disclosure

Whether or not a lesbian or gay man chooses to come out has consequences for their health. Disclosure is often considered to bring benefits while non-disclosure only brings risks. There are, however, benefits and risks in both decisions. The risks of non-disclosure are that health may be negatively affected: lesbians and gay men who hide their sexual identity may be subject to inappropriate questioning, inaccurate diagnoses, irrelevant health information and they may experience anxiety about inadvertently revealing (or avoiding questions about) their sexual identity in the health encounter.

Disclosure on the other hand is seen to be associated with health benefits; lesbians and gay men are likely to be more satisfied and comfortable with the care they receive, they experience greater ease in communicating with their doctor, and by disclosing, they allow for the possibility of including their same-sex partner in treatment decisions. But the risks of disclosing can be high. They include refusal of care, intimidating health care interactions, breaches of confidentiality, embarrassment and infliction of pain (Stevens, 1995). LGBs were more likely to believe that disclosure would adversely affect their health care than improve it. Research conducted on disclosure has suggested that the positive changes which have occurred in societal attitudes have not extended to health care settings (Eliason and Schope, 2001). In addition, disclosure continues to be linked with personal characteristics (social support, disclosure to others) (Boehmer and Case, 2004).

The culture of medicine is dedicated to identifying the symptoms of ill health. For lesbians and gay men this has been problematic because being a lesbian or a gay man has historically been linked to pathology. Early conceptions of lesbian health placed it within a sickness paradigm; for gay men, their sexual identities were systematically linked to disease throughout the HIV/AIDS pandemic. Infamously, the link was made in the (now repealed) section 28 of the 1988 Local Government Act. There may be good reasons, then, for resisting the association between sexual identity and illness by not disclosing. In fact, some believe they can only receive positive health care if they do not disclose: one gay man believed that passing as heterosexual provided a safeguard against poor treatment (Beehler, 2001).

In this analysis of coming out to health care providers, disclosure and non-disclosure are considered as strategies of resistance or accommodation to heterosexist normative assumptions. Seven focus groups were conducted with lesbians to explore their health care experiences. I analyse lesbians' talk about coming out and staying in the closet in relation to four strategies proposed by Hitchcock and Wilson (1992): active non-disclosure (claiming an assumed identity); passive non-disclosure (hiding or avoiding questions about one's sexual identity); passive disclosure (giving clues about sexual identity); and active disclosure (directly telling a health professional about one's sexual identity). I go on to consider two issues which influence disclosure and non-disclosure: the heterosexual presumption and the relevance of sexual identity to health care. While this analysis may be limited by seeming to propose four mutually exclusive strategies for disclosure, rather than fluid and overlapping positions, it does avoid the constraints of the dichotomous model.

Active non-disclosure

When a lesbian chooses not to disclose to a health professional she is said to deliberately present herself as heterosexual. Active non-disclosure is associated with the identity management strategies of closeted lesbians. It is said to resemble a masquerade or a charade; consequently, hiding one's sexual identity, may not be something that many lesbian, gay and bisexual people would want to admit to doing. Although 28 per cent of lesbians in a previous study had not disclosed to their health professional, none had claimed a heterosexual identity or actively concealed their sexual identity (Boehmer and Case, 2004). By contrast, in this study, lesbians provided accounts where they actively decided not to disclose or intentionally misled their health professional. There were three circumstances in the focus groups where lesbians chose, or were obliged to adopt, active non-disclosure: (1) concerns about confidentiality, (2) contraception and (3) hospital visiting rights. Confidentiality is an issue for Donna who is concerned that her identity as a lesbian mother will be written on her newborn daughter's medical notes:

Extract 1

Sonya: For me there's no difference between erm lesbians or straight women, I think women get a bad deal.

Kate: I think the difference would be if you have problems being out in that situation with that medical person.

Donna: I think it kind of says something that when I was having my child and I was going to go to the hospital some friends who are gay said to me for God's sake when they ask you who the

father is say you don't know, because it's better that you're
labelled a slag than a lesbian . . .

Laura: What did you decide in the end?

Donna: I just never told them anything, they didn't ask. I did do one
lie. And I feel a bit bad about that when they asked if I was
in a stable relationship I said no. Because I knew they were
going to assume it was a man.

Sonya says there are no differences in the experiences of lesbians and
heterosexual women and this prompts an exploration among participants about different health care experiences. The example above is
interesting insofar as the decision to 'tell a lie' about her sexual identity
was not a private decision made between Donna and her partner, but
one that was advocated by a group of lesbian friends. It disrupts notions
that those who have social support from other lesbians are more likely
to come out than those who are socially isolated. It may be that her
description of her friends as gay (women), rather than lesbians, is indica-
tive of their political affiliations; nonetheless Donna uses the word 'lesbian' elsewhere in the extract.

In the following extract, Bev is asked about her needs for contraception during her smear test. She elects to pass as heterosexual by asking
for (and being given) contraception that she does not need rather than
disclose her sexual identity:

Extract 2

Bev: And that's always a shocker isn't it? When they say 'what
            form of contraception do you use?'

Karen: I've heard that one before.

Bev: Yes that's always an embarrassing one isn't it?

Facilitator: What do you usually do?

Bev: Give us a bag of condoms.

Even though the conversation implies that the question about contraception is a common, everyday experience, in the use of 'always', 'I've heard
that one before' and 'usually', Bev reacts to the question with shock and
embarrassment. In contrast to the first extract, there is a sense of surprise, rather than pre-planning, in the response. Bev has not made a verbal statement – I am heterosexual – but by asking for condoms, she has
promoted that assumption.

Kathy needs to visit her partner in hospital; however, she is granted conditional visiting rights:

Extract 3

Kathy: My ex-partner had a radical hysterectomy last year for cervical cancer and the issue around that was access. I think that's a big issue for lesbians if your partner's in hospital.

Tracey: Yes.

Kathy: Who are you? What I was, was the sister. I mean everybody on the ward knew, or probably knew, that I was her partner what the nurse in charge said was say you're her sister.

Barbara: God you're joking.

Kathy: They allowed me complete access at any time of the day or night, they were great but . . .

Tracey: Only if you said you were her sister.

In active non-disclosure lesbians take steps to conceal and keep secret their sexual identity; they provide 'false' clues about themselves which are likely to be interpreted as indicating heterosexuality. Active non-disclosure is sometimes the result of a thought-out strategy which may involve some form of pretence (Donna talks about telling one lie, Kathy goes on to suggest that it was an open secret). In these extracts, lesbians assume a range of identities: promiscuous woman, sexually active heterosexual woman, and sister. In the first two extracts, active non-disclosure is a strategy of accommodation adopted by the two women themselves; in the third, however, active non-disclosure is imposed on Kathy. The charge nurse implies that Kathy's access to her partner relies upon pretending to be a sibling: the inference is that a sister is a valued and recognised relationship which merits visiting rights.

Lesbians who choose active non-disclosure are commonly believed to lack the support of family and friends and are closeted in other areas of their lives. But in subsequent discussion, each of them provided examples of being out; for example, Donna described being open to the nursery workers in her rural community. Moreover, two of them had been involved in lesbian and gay activism.

Passive non-disclosure

In passive non-disclosure, a lesbian does not claim a different identity (as in active non-disclosure), but neither does she give clues about her identity (as in passive disclosure). Instead she hides, remains invisible, manages her appearance and passes as heterosexual by avoiding questions which would oblige her to disclose, or she fails to correct mistaken assumptions about her sexual identity. It is often seen to be an omission, rather than an active decision. Three circumstances in which lesbians chose passive non-disclosure were (1) questions about sexual history and contraception, (2) hospital waiting room, and (3) the use of the speculum. Although I have categorised the first extract as passive non-disclosure – because a heterosexual identity has not been actively claimed – Alison resists disclosure in the face of persistent questions about her sexual behaviour. She refuses to disclose, but she does not claim to be heterosexual:

Extract 4

Alison: When I changed doctors 15 months ago the first thing they did was gave me a questionnaire and said [inaudible] erm then I had to see the nurse she said I must just ask you are you in a regular relationship with a man, I kind of laughed hysterically and said no and she said what contraception do you use? No. She said are you on the pill. I said no. She said do you use condoms? I said no. She said well when you are in a relationship, do you use condoms? No. I was nearly on the floor by that point and I wasn't sure whether to tell her I was a lesbian or not because there's just no provision for it on the form at all.

Even though Alison responds to questions five times with a negative, it appears that the practice nurse still did not consider the possibility that Alison might be lesbian. Her questions may be unconscious and unintentional, but their effect is far from benign. Alison says that she laughed hysterically at the questions and was almost on the floor. It is not surprising that Alison chose not to disclose in such an encounter; the barrage of questions and the practice nurse's failure to pick up on Alison's feelings suggest that she would not receive a positive response. The extract suggests not only that the practice nurse appears to be particularly unlikely to consider the possibility of an alternative to heterosexuality, but also the sexual history taking forms do not allow for lesbianism. As Ponse (1978) contends, conversations which are relatively matter-of-fact for heterosexual people may occasion elaborate impression management for the non-disclosed lesbian – a further example is provided below. The extract provides an illustration about the ways heterosexist assumptions operate and might explain how the director of the UK National Cervical Screening Programme can say that women are not asked about their sexual behaviour and lesbians say that they *are* asked. There may be other issues at play here, about the inter-relationship between sexual identity and other identities. Alison identifies as a disabled lesbian. There were no other examples in the data where lesbians were asked the specific question: Are you in a regular relationship with a man?

Karen has been referred for a diagnostic mammogram; she describes her experience in the hospital waiting room:

Extract 5

Karen: Going to hospital was a strange experience, sitting there with your basket and making sure you don't stick out, trying not to look too much like a dyke so that you make everyone else feel uncomfortable [laughter] looking down here so that you're not looking at anybody.

Karen did not manage her appearance to conform to heterosexual femininity, but neither did she want to draw attention to herself or offend the sensitivities of others by her appearance. Heterosexuals often appear to be offended by anything other than the disguised performance of homosexuality. Karen evidently felt that she looked visibly lesbian and tried to manage the discomfort of others by not looking people in the eye, a gesture which might be considered passive (and thus not typically associated with lesbians). Looking down can be interpreted as a marker of stereotypical, heterosexual femininity.

In the next extract, Robyn, in common with some other lesbians, prefers to have the smallest-sized speculum when she attends for a smear test. Because smaller specula are linked with women who have never had vaginal intercourse, Robyn's request might be interpreted as a (somewhat obscure) clue to her sexual identity. She does not confirm, or deny, this association:

Extract 6

Robyn: No if I go for a smear I always ask for the smallest possible – whatever it is they stick up you [the speculum] – you know, I usually ask for the child's one. But I don't tell them why.

Lesbians often face the decision of whether to come out when they attend for cervical screening, particularly at a new surgery where it is usual practice for a sexual history to be taken. In passive non-disclosure, lesbians avoid answering such questions in ways which would reveal their sexual identity. Their behaviour is passive insofar as they do not mislead, but in many respects the word passive is a misnomer. Alison actively resists disclosing her identity in the face of what can only be described as an interrogation. In the survey, lesbians also described the questioning for the sexual history as *intrusive, awkward, insensitive, irrelevant, difficult*; but also the style of questioning was *inappropriate, interrogative*; or the health care provider *absolutely grilled me* by asking *the usual questions*, as well as lots of them.

Accommodating to the closet is not a simple, effortless act (Seidman, 2002). It involves the deliberate management of oneself, others and situations. Lesbians who 'pass' are concerned to conceal their lesbian identity and present a convincing heterosexual front to straight audiences. In order to 'pass' successfully, they must develop a heightened awareness of everyday encounters. At times, lesbians, gay men and bisexuals engage in elaborate self-protective routines based on cultural assumptions of heterosexuality which involve constant monitoring of topics of conversation, and the management of one's appearance or behaviour (Hughes, 2004). At other times, lesbians, gay men and bisexuals have to do comparatively little to avoid detection, although this can also be a choice about how one's sexual identity is presented – in one's clothes, styles of walking and talking.

Passive disclosure

In passive disclosure, lesbians give clues about their sexual identity and allow the health professional to decipher the meaning. In the following extract, Jo and Gill are partners discussing whether their GP knows they are lesbian. They live at the same address and are registered with the same GP and these could be sufficient reasons for believing that their GP is aware about the nature of their relationship. Furthermore, their GP had recently made a number of home visits during an illness of Gill's mother who was living with them at the time. Although it is not inevitable that their GP will know they are lesbians (two women living together are often seen as less remarkable than two men in the same position), they both agree that it is probable that he will know. It raises questions about the quality of knowing: When does someone know? What information does a lesbian need to divulge about her identity? How might that information be communicated? In the extract below, Jo has already come out to a doctor in a hospital setting, but she does not know if the medical notes were passed to the GP, or indeed whether her sexual identity was recorded in her notes. This exemplifies the nature of passive disclosure in particular (although it is also true for the other strategies to a greater or lesser degree): knowledge about sexual identity is highly ambivalent. It is often not clear whether or not someone knows about one's sexual identity.

Extract 7

Facilitator: Do your GPs by and large know that you're lesbian?
Gill: [makes noise] Well Dr Elliott might do.
Jo: Yes. Actually I think the one that dealt with Gill's mum would do.
Gill: But the others don't.
Jo: The others don't, but I don't think it would . . .
Gill: The practice nurses don't either.
Jo: No. But I think he would and he's the one that I go and see, and he's fine.
Gill: But the nurses that do the smear tests.
Jo: Not unless it was put on my records after my trip into hospital.
Gill: They probably do then.
Robyn: But nobody ever reads your records. So it don't matter.
Jo: So no. It's never made [pause] if I was asked I would tell them. But I've never been asked.

Jo had previously come out to a hospital doctor and does not know whether this information has been recorded in her medical notes. If her sexual identity was recorded, then all the staff at her GP surgery might have access to this information. Even though it is probable that the GP knows about their sexual identities because of his visits to their home, both Gill and Jo do not assume that he will have told other professionals at the GP practice. (However, participants in other studies say that a reason for non-disclosure to health professionals is the probability that they would become the subject of social gossip and anecdotal evidence suggests that one's identity is the first piece of information that is communicated about LGB people.) Jo also indicates a willingness to divulge her sexual identity if requested. Many lesbians appear to prefer not to volunteer information about their sexual identity, but would not deny being lesbian if directly asked. Coming out is often misunderstood by some heterosexual people who view it as flaunting or revealing personal information inappropriately. It may mean that some lesbians are reluctant to put their lesbianism into words. But it is also a feature of heterosexism that many LGB people tacitly recognise that access to services is allowed provided that they keep their sexual identity secret. This assumption is the basis of the US military policy: *Don't ask, Don't tell.*

The following extract is taken from qualitative data in the survey; because written data obscure the emphasis placed on words, it is not wholly clear whether the survey participant intended to disclose her identity:

Extract 8

I was asked when I last had sex – I said my last experience of penetrative sex with a man was nine years ago – she said never mind, I'm sure you'll find someone soon. With an instrument in place and my legs at 10 to 2 I didn't feel comfortable telling her I was a lesbian!

The deliberateness of the response – of spelling out the time-scale since she last had heterosexual sex and the kind of sex she had (penetrative) – seems to invite further questions. (It may also be an example of the difficulties lesbians have in meanings about sex discussed in Chapter 4.) Instead, the practice nurse dismisses the nine years as a period of celibacy. Lesbians sometimes disclose their identities in subtle ways, but the opportunity presented to discuss this further was not taken by the practice nurse.

Passive disclosure occurs when lesbians and gay men drop hints and clues about their identity which allow heterosexuals and sometimes other lesbians and gay men to draw inferences about their identity without denying or confirming them. In passive disclosure, nothing is said explicitly and it is often ambiguous whether or not the health care provider has understood the clues given or whether they have read the medical notes. Ponse (1978) describes such disclosures as counterfeit secrecy; others suggest that a fiction is maintained. The first extract conveys some of the ambiguities surrounding partial disclosures – of not knowing who knows – while the second illustrates some of the obstacles to disclosure.

Active disclosure

A critical feature in many accounts of disclosure is the verbal assertion of sexual identity; in many ways, it is the definitive coming out strategy. According to Ponse (1978), putting one's gayness into words marks the irrevocable breaking of secrecy; behaviours and situations are capable of multiple interpretations, but words are not. In the focus groups, however, there were relatively few occasions in which lesbians made the unequivocal statement: 'I am a lesbian.' Many instances of active disclosure contained the neutral 'my partner' followed by the gender-specific pronoun, in this case, 'she' or the use of the partner's name in a context which confirmed the relationship. Nevertheless, in active disclosure, lesbians and gay men explicitly tell their GP or other provider about their sexual identity.

The following extract is interesting because three different experiences and approaches to disclosure are described. Nicky describes herself as a gay woman who has been out to everyone from the age of twenty. In this extract, she provides an example of a clear and unequivocal statement:

Extract 9

Olivia: It gets worse anyway no, no I get it every time. Every – single – time I go in and I've had 3 or 4 now? Every time I go in they ask me exactly the same questions.

Jo: The only questions, the only questions they ask me are: am I sexually active 'yes' am I on the pill 'no'.

Nicky: I've never had that.

Olivia: Oh I get more than that.

Jo: And that's virtually the questions I have so, and they don't say well do you have, have you had a boyfriend or are you married or anything like that.

Robyn: It depends which surgery you go to.

Nicky: Because I'm gay . . .

Olivia: I get [pause] when was the last time? I remember . . .

Nicky: I just avoid all that, they start asking me those questions I say look I'm gay.

Jo: But they still ask you if you're sexually active or if you're on the pill.

Nicky: No, the first question they ask is are you sexually active? and you say 'yes', are you on the pill? 'no' and I just pre-empt it then and say look to save further questions I'm gay.

Nicky's approach to active disclosure is matter-of-fact, emphasised in her calm repetition of the phrase 'I'm gay'. Her reasons for disclosing are to avoid the persistent questioning about her sexual behaviour and contraception needs. Nicky has demanded change in an environment that oppresses her.

In Extract 10, Laura also uses disclosure to actively subvert heterosexist assumptions:

Extract 10

Laura: It's almost worth telling them just to see the fluster isn't it?
Terry: Absolutely.
Ginny: I've done that.
Terry: Just to see what happens.
Laura: I've had so much [pause] when I felt strong enough and the occasion's been right it's quite sadistic, but . . .
Donna: Yeah, always worth it.
Laura: About the only rank I can pull.

Laura says she pulled rank by coming out to her GP. Of course, pulling rank is not about asserting the superiority of homosexuality over heterosexuality, but a way of resisting the authority invested in the health professional and asserting some control in the health care interaction. Here the shock and embarrassment – referred to in Extract 2 which was experienced by a lesbian who did not disclose – is experienced by the health professional instead. Two issues appear to influence Laura's decision to disclose: her own feelings of emotional strength and her ability to choose the timing of disclosure. Her strategy receives confirmation from other focus group members; Terry provides a motivation for such a strategy – to see how the health professional might react. In contrast to Extract 1, where Donna adopted active non-disclosure, here she says that it is *always* worth disclosing. The apparent discontinuity is interesting; in theory lesbians may value being out, in practice they may find it is not always possible.

In Extract 11, Olivia says that when she attends for cervical screening, she feels intimidated by questions about sexual behaviour:

Extract 11

Olivia: Do you ever feel sort of erm you know when you're going for the check and the nurse is there and they ask you sort of are you having regular sex and all that sort of do you ever feel really intimidated by that?
Jo: No.
Robyn: I think it's hilarious. I can't wait for them to ask.

Gill: [laughs] I've never been asked that question.
Jo: Yes they have, because they said to you, you're really clean in there and you said yes I have a woman in twice a day.

[Laughter]

This extract is probably not an example of disclosure, but rather humour in the coming out event. There are few examples in the literature of the comedic possibilities in disclosure; humour is another strategy in claiming control.

There were no examples, as in the US literature, of lesbians coming out to a GP at the initial consultation in order to ascertain the doctor's attitudes towards sexual identity. But this may be an outcome of a different health care system: choice of doctor has been less possible in the UK. Active disclosure is a strategy of resistance to heterosexual domination (Seidman, 2002) and is used to put a stop to persistent questioning or to assert control in the interaction. By refusing to remain silent and invisible, lesbians, gay men and bisexuals challenge heterosexual privilege. Regular disclosure diminishes the secret quality of sexual minority identities; it is liberating and legitimating. Disclosure is said to improve physical health and mental well-being; whether or not a lesbian is able to disclose is an important factor in her experience of health care. Active disclosure may elicit three possible reactions from health care providers: acceptance, neutrality or rejection; these are explored in Chapter 7.

The heterosexual presumption

The heterosexual presumption works in a number of ways in relation to disclosure and non-disclosure. It often allows lesbians to pass as heterosexual in health care encounters (e.g. Donna in Extract 1 and Bev in Extract 2), but it also imposes heterosexuality (for Kathy in Extract 3) or prevents disclosure (for Alison in Extract 4). One of the reasons given, for coming out to their health care provider, in the extracts of active disclosure is that lesbians will avoid unnecessary questions in the future. There have been similar findings elsewhere. But lesbians who make unequivocal statements as Nicky has done cannot always assume this means that they will not face heterosexual assumptions:

Extract 12

Even though this doctor knew I was a lesbian, he still kept making inane conversation about heterosexual topics. Like he tried to joke with me about boyfriends. Then he got silent. Then it was like he forgot, and he started to flirt with me. Then he hesitated. He was obviously uncomfortable and he was stumped for how to make conversation with me. (Stevens, 1995: 28)

Here, the heterosexual presumption prescribes how men and women relate to each other; because lesbians do not fit into this matrix, some people do not 'know how to behave or what to say to them' (Markowe, 1996: 144). The doctor jokes, flirts and makes inane conversation because he seems not to know how to relate to women otherwise. There were other examples in the data where lesbians had disclosed to their health professionals and were still asked what contraception they were using. Coming out is not necessarily a guarantee against inappropriate questions or interactions.

Relevance of sexual identity to health care

Particular health problems, such as those relating to sexual behaviour or mental health, are considered more relevant to one's sexual identity than others. The relevance of one's sexual identity to the health problem is said to be more likely to prompt disclosure. Lack of relevance is the most common reason for non-disclosure and, in one study, more than two-thirds of participants said that their sexual identity was not relevant to their most recent health care visit (Eliason and Schope, 2001). Sexual identity is considered of less (or no) relevance for some health care needs, such as obtaining a mammogram.

For some, disclosure can only occur if there are compelling reasons. Does the health care provider 'need to know'? In the following extract, a lesbian considers whether disclosure makes sense, as she develops her argument, she finds there are many more reasons to disclose than she had first thought:

Extract 13

I would disclose only if it made sense. Like I needed therapy, or if I had a debilitating illness and I was going to need lots of care, or if I was being hospitalized and I wanted to make sure my partner could visit, or if I was being tested for HIV, or if I was planning to have a child, or if I really liked a doctor and thought I would be working with her for a long time. (Stevens, 1994: 223)

Her list of the circumstances and health needs for which she might decide to reveal her sexual identity include those which are widely perceived to be relevant such as mental health and sexual behaviour; in addition, she lists situations where her sexual identity is likely to become visible, such as if her partner visited her in hospital. The account, however, continues the link between disclosure and the relevance of certain conditions or circumstances. Relevance did not appear to be associated with disclosure decisions in the extracts considered in this chapter, despite the fact that the circumstances in some of them were those most linked to relevance in other studies. Donna did not come out as a lesbian mother-to-be, nor did Bev reveal that she had no need for contraception. By contrast, in a situation apparently unconnected to relevance, Karen used identity management strategies in an attempt to avoid attention (Extract 5).

In the following extract, Sarah suggests that even for a health problem as mundane and (apparently) unrelated to sexual identity as an inflamed stomach, her lesbianism is indeed relevant. Being out facilitates open discussion:

Extract 14

Sarah: The first time you walk in the door under any circumstances . . . nine times out of ten – unless you're going in for a cold – it seems you will talk about something to do with your home life and recently I had . . . an inflamed stomach. They gave me some antacid and it was really painful. I was talking about my eating habits and when you talk about your eating habits, anyone else would say we have this or we have that. Well anyway, I can't remember exactly what I said and I knew she knew my situation it was just much easier.

Irene: So you could say the food that Irene cooks is . . .

Sarah: What made me ill. I don't think I did, but you just feel comfortable talking about your whole circumstances, life and everything else and you need to when you're seeing your GP even if it is only about what your diet and exercise is.

Overwhelmingly in the literature, sexual identity is considered most relevant when heterosexuality is routinely assumed: in sexual history taking, sexually transmitted diseases and contraception. In these circumstances, disclosure is said to be important information for health care providers because it facilitates accurate diagnoses and appropriate treatment (Eliason and Schope, 2001). But the notion of relevance needs to be problematised because it reinscribes a biomedical approach to lesbians' and gay men's health. By using the concept of relevance, we perpetuate an illness-specific approach to health. The assumption that health care providers only need to know about sexual identity in order to provide an accurate diagnosis continues this dependence on a biomedical approach to health. Health professionals need to know about sexual identity in order to provide holistic health care: not just a quick diagnosis. By using relevance as a marker for disclosure, however, we may be unwittingly perpetuating some of the heterosexist views about lesbians and gay men that we are in fact seeking to challenge. Western medicine does not treat the whole person, only the part that is sick. The medical model separates our bodies into discrete units demonstrated in the specialties: cardiac, obstetrics, ear, nose and throat, and so on. Beliefs about relevance reinforce the notion that our identity is located only in relation to some aspects of our health, for example, sexual health, even though lesbians have challenged the notion of our identities being located only in sex.

By applying the concept of relevance to heterosexual identities, its underlying heterosexism is revealed. A possible parallel might be to consider whether one would want (if it were possible) to separate other identities in this way. If you were to ask a heterosexual man whether his heterosexuality was relevant to his most recent health care visit or whether he should disclose it, he is likely to say it is not relevant. Yet heterosexual men are commonly less exposed to the indicators of ill health: they earn more in comparison to heterosexual women doing similar work with equivalent skills and qualifications, they tend to have more leisure time and spend less time doing housework and related tasks. If he were accidentally to let slip that he was in a relationship with a woman, his GP is unlikely to show much consternation, nor to make certain assumptions about his sexual behaviour. Nor is his GP likely to assume that his heterosexuality is the cause of his health problem even if the problem was of a genito-urinary nature. His health is privileged in innumerable ways by his heterosexuality, but his heterosexuality is seen to bear no relationship to his well-being. The concept of relevance, then, only applies to LGB identities and never to heterosexual identities. It continues the assumption that LGB identities can somehow become detached from core identities and that being a lesbian or a gay man is only related to sexual or mental health problems. This compartmentalisation is evident in other circumstances; for example, where lesbians do not disclose because they wish to avoid being known as a lesbian rather than oneself (Markowe, 1996).

How have the focus groups contributed to knowledge about the closet and coming out?

The use of focus groups gave participants the opportunity to discursively explore the continua of disclosure and non-disclosure; they were not obliged to make a categorical yes/no statement. Often these narratives of disclosure and non-disclosure occurred in the context of a general discussion about health care, rather than in response to a specific question: Are you out to your GP? Unlike one-to-one interviews where lesbians seem reluctant to say they are closeted, here, lesbians talked about actively and passively remaining in the closet. At times, they intentionally misled health professionals about their sexual identity and failed to correct mistaken assumptions. But they also used a range of strategies to signal their sexual identity to their health providers, including direct statements.

As method, focus groups enable participants to identify their own perspectives and priorities. They can discuss, disagree or confirm their perceptions with others with similar or different experiences. While group discussion does not allow the researcher to quantify how many of the participants were out and to whom, it does produce useful insights about the experiences of coming out and being closeted. The stories lend testimony to the difficulties in both disclosure and non-disclosure. Lesbians described being uncomfortable, intimidated, embarrassed, hysterical, as well as feeling a bit bad (because she lied). They provided examples of conditional access, a strange experience, and questioning that got worse with each visit. At times, being out and being closeted were fraught experiences.

Coming out is often seen as a once-only event typified by the Ellen DeGeneres experience. But in these accounts of coming out, lesbians described a continual decision-making process about whether or not to disclose, how to disclose or whether their sexual identity is already known. Even the few lesbians who said they were out in all aspects of their lives, might have to deal with interactions that assume heterosexuality as described in Extract 12. The focus group narratives of disclosure and non-disclosure speak of episodic patterns of concealment rather than the prison or geography which have characterised earlier representations. They are actively defended positions even when they are categorised as passive; for the most part, they are situation-contingent occasions in which lesbians were sometimes closeted and sometimes out.

It might be that at the beginning of the twenty-first century there are fewer LGB people who live in complete isolation than in previous decades. These narratives suggest that lesbians who remain closeted are not necessarily more socially isolated than those who do come out. If lesbians are not out in a health care setting, they may well be out in other areas of their lives. In one of the focus groups, participants discuss the level of support recently offered to a lesbian within their social circle with breast cancer. This friendship group, of which they were all members, included approximately 80 lesbians who did not live in a large city:

Extract 15

Olivia: When something goes wrong everybody closes ranks.
Nicky: Yes.
Olivia: And I think because of the nature of the group itself then that has a big effect on people.
Jo: I mean we have discos and dos we all come together and know one another, we're all gay. You don't get that in the heterosexual world. You don't get everybody being friends because they're heterosexual, you get people being friends because they've yes . . .
Robyn: Worked together.
Jo: Because they've worked together or they're neighbours or they've grown up together or they've been school buddies together so you get, it's not-the-same I don't think.

Being out describes a valued status: individuals who are out have rebelled against the closet, they are 'active, thoughtful, risk-takers'; those who are closeted are passive victims who 'surrender to things as they are' (Seidman, 2002: 31). The continued association of the closet with passive and lonely individuals suggests that the closet is only inhabited by the socially iso-lated and has little applicability to the lives of the majority of LGB peo-ple. The characterisation of those who do not disclose as passive victims continues an individualised, psychological approach which blames LGB people for their decisions. We see it as the problem the individual has with being out (as Kate does in Extract 1) instead of a heterosexist envi-ronment which places limits on disclosure. As Robinson (1997) argues, we risk blaming LGB people for contributing to their oppression and often wrongly assume that liberating choices are always available to them. By suggesting that the closet is only a feature in the lives of a small number of isolated individuals, we ignore how it continues to be a life-shaping presence even among the most forthright.

7
Screened Out: Lesbians' Experiences of Cervical Screening

Relationships with health care professionals

The relationship between health professionals (especially doctors) and women patients has been a popular topic for study in medical sociology over a number of years. Feminists have analysed the relationship as a site of power and control where doctors are in positions of institutional authority. Sociologists have shown that socially excluded groups, especially working class and black women, have differentiated experiences of health care. Black and working class women are less likely to participate in cervical screening because of poor explanations and because professionals operate in a culture of silence (Chiu and Knight, 1999). Lesbians are also less likely to attend for cervical screening, but they are overlooked in government targets to promote uptake. Research has suggested that most GPs were not aware they had any lesbian patients, despite many years in practice. Few knew of relevant health issues for lesbians or had ever asked about sexual identity. A recent study found that sexual identity formed a barrier to discussion about sexual health matters for almost half the GPs in the sample; difficulties related to ignorance of lesbian and gay lifestyles and homophobic attitudes were identified among a minority (Hinchliff et al., 2005).

Lesbians' experiences of health care

Lesbians' experiences of health care have been extensively researched in relation to a range of health care disciplines; more recently, a smaller body of work has considered gay men's experiences of primary care (Cant, 1999; Beehler, 2001; Keogh et al., 2004b). While there may be a number of similarities between their experiences, this chapter focuses on lesbians' experiences of health care and their interactions with health professionals. Throughout the lesbian health literature, researchers have found that lesbians do not access a range of service provision because of their adverse experiences of health care or because of their knowledge of the experiences of others, including partners and friends (Scherzer, 2000). Previous studies have found that lesbians were obliged to negotiate a range of barriers to good care, including ignorance of their needs and moral disapproval (Wilton and Kaufmann, 2001). Further examination of the nature of these experiences reveals that professionals lack knowledge about lesbians' health needs and, in particular, their risks for cervical cancer; lesbians are reluctant to place themselves in situations where they may be obliged to disclose their sexual identity; they anticipate a heterosexist reaction from health professionals; and lesbians themselves believe they are at low risk for cervical cancer (retrieved 11 August 2005 from http://www.cdc.gov/ncidod/EID/vol10no11/04-0467.htm). Adverse experiences can have a number of far-reaching consequences beyond the circumstances in which they occur: they are said to affect subsequent rates of attendance, make future examinations more difficult and lead to poor health outcomes.

By comparison, the literature about lesbians' positive experiences of health care is less developed. Many researchers have emphasised that the interaction between a health professional and patient is central to the provision of positively perceived health care and the attitudes of health care workers towards lesbians have a major impact on the care that they receive. Studies have revealed that lesbians prefer a female health professional particularly for intimate examinations such as smear tests. Lesbians rate their care as good when their partners are included in treatment and decision-making. Professionals who created an environment where it was safe to disclose were also valued. Knowing about lesbians' good experiences may aid the development of effective health interventions.

The literature suggests that lesbians are more likely to report adverse, rather than positive, experiences of health – even among recent studies, heterosexist attitudes towards lesbians and gay men are in evidence. Cervical screening has emerged as a key area of health inequality for lesbians: their reduced frequency of attendance and their risk factors for the disease are now understood. While lesbians' experiences of health, particularly in relation to primary care have been investigated (Stevens, 1998), less is known specifically about lesbians' experiences when the smear test is taken. Yet gynaecological care is believed to cause more distress to lesbians because of the physical and emotional vulnerability it entails (Scherzer, 2000). Moreover, previous studies have been small-scale and qualitative; while they have investigated the nature of lesbians' health care interactions, they do not tell us how far these experiences are shared by lesbians. The

Table 7.1:   Lesbians' screening experiences

Screening experiences	Positive		Adverse	
	%	N	%	N
Attitudes and behaviour of health professionals	38	311	25	194
Aspects of the procedure	36	291	31	245
Pain-free or painful experiences	16	128	39	308
Other explanations	10	84	5	40
Totals	100	814	100	787

LHCS focused on lesbians' experiences of screening and it is unusual because it elicited qualitative explanations from 1066 lesbians. It enables the combination of qualitative and quantitative data to provide insight into the nature of lesbians' screening experiences: whether there are particular issues in the way in which the smear test is performed and how common those experiences are.

How the study was carried out

In the LHCS, lesbians were asked two questions about their experiences of smear tests. Of the 901 lesbians who had attended for smear tests, 46 per cent (N = 418, of 901) reported positive experiences and 44 per cent (N = 394, of 901) reported adverse ones. Both questions included a text box where lesbians could give reasons for their evaluations. Analysis revealed three major themes for their screening experiences and these are presented in Table 7.1.

Attitudes and behaviour of health professionals

Poor explanations

The inappropriate attitudes and behaviour of health professionals were cited in a quarter of reasons for adverse experiences of smear tests. Lesbians said that the health professional did not explain the procedure and they did not know what to expect – this was particularly important for the first test: *the first time I had one nothing was explained to me what they would do & why they were doing it. Or what 'that speculum thing' was that they had just taken out of the drawer + were running under the tap!!* Others stated that the health care worker did not offer reassurance or help them to relax; in other interactions, lesbians were ignored: *and constantly spoke to a colleague during it, without even interacting with me in any way.* Lesbians reported that practitioners were *abrupt; unsympathetic; impatient; really patronising; rude; uncommunicative* and *impersonal*. They recounted experiences of routine treatment: *insensitive people just doing their job no care for client = client made to feel like a number NOT A* PERSON [sic]*; In a GUM clinic I felt like a piece of meat on a conveyor belt.* Others were blamed: *Told to relax! Implication was it was my fault for not being relaxed – for it hurting.* Sometimes this disapprobation was quite subtle: *I don't think this is anyone's fault but I have been left with the feeling that the failure of the smears has been down to my bodily failure e.g. I've put on weight – my uterus is tilted etc; I left feeling very put off by the experience – sense of being 'useless' + somehow criticised.*

Heterosexist assumptions

The assumption of heterosexuality is routine and pervasive in health (and social care) interactions. In their descriptions of adverse experiences, lesbians said that health professionals exhibited heterosexist attitudes and behaviour. Heterosexuality is routinely assumed in *inappropriate* or *intrusive questions asked about my birth control needs despite my assurances that I don't need any; assumption of heterosexual sex by nurses* or by the environment in which a smear takes place: *Couldn't explain I was a dyke, though I tried. The whole clinic was totally hetero.* The presumption of heterosexuality can sometimes mean that a lesbian is unable to 'come out':

> The practice nurse assumed as I was heterosexual and started asking what contraception I used. When I said none she once again assumed that I was sexually inactive and rather abruptly told me that 'I shouldn't be having one then'. Her attitude was rather grudging that she should be giving me a smear, her tone patronising, making me feel that I'd wasted her time. I didn't feel able to tell her that I was a lesbian.

On other occasions a lesbian may decide to 'come out' to stop the questions: *Doctor with hand inside me asking insistently – if I could be pregnant when I'd last had a period and sex, if I had a partner, if I used contraception until I came out to him to shut him up – (it did).* Some stated that health care workers were very uncomfortable in performing a smear for a lesbian: *even now I think sometimes straight women are freaked out about doing one on an out dyke.* Some lesbians said that they had a heterosexist response when they did come out to the health care worker: *I mentioned my girlfriend to the nurse, and she bolted – and got a male nurse to come and do it.* Or their confidentiality was breached in their medical notes: *nurse read on notes that I was gay and insisted on being accompanied by another person.* Some lesbians reported that they were refused smears. This refusal was made in a number of ways, for example, by negating the 'validity' of lesbian sexuality: *She said that having sex with women did not count – I was not sexually active and therefore didn't really need a smear.* Or by equating lesbian sex with virginity:

> student health care centre AnyCity. The nurse doing the pre-weighing + pre-questioning etc. asked what contraception I used. When I said I was Lesbian she shouted (so all outside could hear) 'So you're a virgin, well she won't be able to do the test' and was horrible when I said I knew the doctor would have no problem she looked at me in disgust – the doctor was OK.

Yet others were told that by having a smear, lesbians would be wasting NHS resources: *As a young lesbian being treated by a male doctor who was blatently* [sic] *homophobic saying as I was not what was classed as sexually active this process was a waste of time and money.* Finally, lesbians reported being viewed as an object of curiosity: *Without my consent, about fifteen students, mostly male, came into the room whilst I was strapped up – presumably to look at a lesbian's cervix!!*

Good relationships with health professionals

When lesbians talked about positive experiences of smear tests, they most frequently referred to health professionals' social skills. The ability of the health provider to establish a good relationship was particularly valued by lesbians in this study. They commented that practitioners helped to reduce their anxiety by creating an atmosphere in which they could 'relax' or they were put 'at ease'. In their descriptions of these relationships, lesbians said that health care workers were: *friendly; sensitive; professional; sympathetic; understanding; positive* and they treated them with *respect*.

Health professionals who provided explanations of what was going to happen contributed to reducing the power imbalance in the relationship: *Carried out by actual GP and she explained procedure step by step; Nurse talking through – explaining the process.* Moreover, lesbians said they had autonomy in the screening process and their previous experiences were not discounted: *I was able to explain to the doctor how I'd felt about the last one; the GP . . . listened to what I said about the previous test . . . I felt . . . that my experience was not being ignored.* Health professionals are often positioned as the experts in medical interventions, knowing more about women's bodies than they do themselves. Practitioners who listened to the information lesbians provided about their bodies were valued: *Careful GP . . . listened to my description of where my cervix head is*. So too, were GPs who were prepared to discuss their health with them.

The absence of heterosexism

In their estimations of positive attitudes and behaviours, lesbians said that the absence of heterosexism made the experience a good one. This was commonly evident in the way in which questions were asked and assumptions were made: *the lack of any intrusive questioning re reasons for non use of contraception!*; *the questions she asked me before the test were not presumtious* [sic] *– she assumed nothing about my sexuality*. In some cases, lesbians reported that the atmosphere was generally supportive: *I've always been out to him, because of his positive attitude in general*; *The nurse was understanding to me being a lesbian*. In other accounts, their sexual identity was acknowledged: *My sexuality was respected*; *just nice to be in a lesbian positive environment*. Other lesbians saw the test as a chance to disclose: *It provided an opportunity to come out to my GP!* Yet others said that they were *Fortunate enough to have a lesbian doctor so just that puts me at ease & know* [sic] *that I don't have to deal with any possible homophobia or ignorance*. Lesbians gave examples of a provider-initiated lesbian sensitive service that placed value on lesbians' relationships: *Encouraging partner* [to be] *present*. Finally, what appears to be a particularly lesbian example of a good experience: *I mended the window blind for the practice nurse, which made me feel useful and hence more equal*.

Health care is often said to have more to do with doctors' values and attitudes than with biology or disease. Patients, in general, overwhelmingly rate their health professionals positively and this is more likely to relate to their interpersonal, rather than their clinical, skills. Good interpersonal skills are indicated by building rapport with a patient and establishing trust. While these issues are important for all patients, they appear to be particularly relevant for lesbians in this study because attitudes and behaviour were the most common explanation given for a positive experience. Moreover, creating an environment safe for disclosure was valued by lesbians. Health professionals can signal acceptance of lesbians by the use of neutral language and by asking open questions about contraceptive needs. They can acknowledge a lesbian's sexual identity and encourage her partner to accompany her for the test. Moreover, displaying a positive attitude in general enables some lesbians to disclose. Other studies have found that lesbians who are open about their identity with their provider are more emotionally healthy, more satisfied with their care, and used preventive care more regularly than women who did not disclose.

Aspects of the procedure

Aspects of the procedure featured in explanations for both adverse and positive experiences of smear tests. Five aspects of the procedure led to an adverse experience, these were: 'gender of health care worker'; 'procedural problems'; 'the speculum'; 'lack of privacy or dignity'; and 'the position for taking the smear'. Three aspects contributed to a positive experience, these were 'issues around taking the smear', 'gender of health care worker', and 'the health care setting for the smear'.

Negative aspects of the procedure

Among reasons for adverse experiences, the most common was the gender of the health care worker. Lesbians said that having a male do the test made the experience unacceptable; this was sometimes because of the attitude he had: *I realised later he wasn't the best person to go to. He really couldn't manage to say 'well woman clinic'*; or because of his conduct: *male doctor took me in a room on my own to do it*; or because the request for a female health care worker was refused: *I had arranged to see a woman doctor for my smear but there was only a male doctor available at the clinic. He was very angry that I tried to insist on seeing a woman doctor. I could have cancelled & come back another day but I was persuaded to go ahead.* Other lesbians said that female health care workers also made the experience a bad one: *Done by practice nurse who would have done better getting a job in an abbatoir* [sic]; or because of their manner: *Last one by a nasty 'matron' type woman.*

Procedural problems also made the test unacceptable. In these explanations, lesbians said that their test had to be repeated for a range of reasons, including: *slide dropped in lab, so had to be repeated; On two occasions* [sic] *I had to go back for further tests in order to get a blood free sample (even though not my period time)*. In lesbians' accounts of the test, the procedure is not straightforward: *test failed; not able to achieve an adequate sample; Insufficient cells were obtained and I had to have the smear redone. This has happened twice.* A number of other lesbians said that the health care worker was only able to find her cervix after several attempts: *last one recently took 5 attempts by 2 different practitioners* or a considerable amount of time: *the student nurse and the GP (woman) couldn't find my cervix (!) and the whole thing took 45 minutes of fumbling and stuff.*

In addition, problems with the speculum were factors in negative aspects of the procedure. In these responses, lesbians talked about the speculum being cold: *The speculum has never been warmed and after the smear my muscles contracted so much that the speculum couldn't be removed without some force*, or occasionally too hot: *I once had a speculum inserted that was too hot! Ow!!* Sometimes the health care worker was aware that the speculum was cold, but nevertheless proceeded with the test: *On one occasion, the nurse said 'normally I warm my hands/instruments, but I haven't the time and I'm going to do this anyway.'* Other lesbians recounted that health care workers did not have different sized specula in their practice rooms, and were indiscreet in asking for an alternative: *The doctor shouted at the nurse to fetch the smallest speculum as I wasn't sexually active*; or left the room to look for one & *she left the big speculum in while she went to look for a smaller one. It's like aversion therapy for healthcare.* Some lesbians stated that a range of specula was used until the correct size was found: *The doctor used the biggest size equipment, which hurt. Then she used the next size down, then the smallest* and others said that despite having asked for a smaller size, their request was ignored: *and regardless how many times you ask for a small speculum, they never believe you until it's too late.*

Lack of privacy or dignity also contributed to an adverse experience. In some cases this was because medical students were present for the test: *The doctor then invited two students (both male) into the room.* In others, however, the room in which the smear is taken appears not to afford privacy: *staff walking in + out.* Some lesbians said there was no recognition of their personal dignity: *Was told by nurse to take my pants off and left for half an hour before the doctor came* or they were left lying on the examination table: *Dr left the 'tool' thing inside me and left the room, leaving me cold and uncomfortable for several minutes.*

Some lesbians said they *dislike intensely the position women are asked to take; typical legs up and away we go.* Others suggest that the position is evocative of heterosex: *Don't like 'missionary position' for smear.*

Positive aspects of the procedure

In relation to positive aspects of the procedure, lesbians most commonly cited issues about the speculum. They mentioned that the speculum had been previously warmed: *The last smear I had the nurse very kindly warmed the instrument before inserting it into me* or that the practice *carries a range of sizes in speculums!* For some lesbians, it was important that the test was conducted *efficiently; quickly* or *was over* before they realised; for others it was important that the health care worker *took their time* or conducted the test at the woman's *own pace.*

Lesbians overwhelmingly said that they preferred to have a female health care worker perform the test. The gender of the health care worker was noted in 100 responses, of which 80 participants said they preferred a woman. A typical response was: *My doctor is a woman & having a woman put her fingers inside me I am quite happy with, although I guess this is just the internal exam & not the smear test.* Some lesbians emphasised that they ensured that a female doctor or nurse conducted the test: *all my smears have been taken by female doctors or nurses. I would not want a male doctor to take one.* A number of lesbians said they valued the choice of who conducted the test or they had an equally good experience from both males and females: *and most of my experiences are that both male and female doctors have treated me with care, respect and sensitivity.* A smaller number reported a preference for a male to perform the test: *by a man doctor, as I feel embarrassed when conducted by a female doctor.*

Lesbians stated that 'the health care setting' for the smear made the experience a good one. This was predominantly because screening took place at one of the lesbian sexual health clinics, which were established almost a decade ago in London, Oxford and Glasgow. These were often mentioned by name and were valued because they provided a service specifically for lesbians: *The staff at the Bernhart* [sic] *clinic are absolutely brilliant as it is specifically for lesbians.* Others said that a well-woman clinic, a GUM clinic or their own GP provided a good service. Yet others were fortunate to have a lesbian GP: *I go to lesbian dr. But she's now part time, & very popular, not just with lesbians, so there's always long waiting list for appointment with her* [sic].

Apart from the gender of the health professional, aspects of the procedure appear to be less discussed in the cervical screening literature. (Presumed) heterosexual women would rather have a woman perform the smear test. Lesbians also find women practitioners to be more sensitive, open to alternative lifestyles and less judgmental than men. But there are also interesting differences between the gender preferences of (presumed) heterosexual women and of lesbians. In one study, 69 per cent of (presumed) heterosexual women preferred a female practitioner, 31 per cent expressed no preference, and none preferred a man. Surprisingly, in the LHCS, of those who expressed a preference for the gender of their health care provider, 80 per cent preferred a woman, 15 per cent said they had no preference and 5 per cent preferred a male. A small number of lesbians stated that the smear test would hold sexual connotations if performed by a woman. Previous research among (presumed) heterosexual women has suggested that the smear is seen as a sexualised encounter; but by their husbands rather than the women themselves.

The health care setting in which the smear is taken has also been found to be a positive aspect of the screening service. In areas of London with low uptake rates, mobile units have been successful in attracting women who have never been screened. (Presumed) heterosexual women are said to value accessibility, proximity and familiarity. By contrast, some lesbians expressed a preference for lesbian sexual health clinics which for many necessitated travelling long distances to attend them.

The speculum is most comfortable when it has been previously warmed; however, some practitioners forget to do this. Women's experiences of cold specula are not generally discussed in the literature. An exception is in a study of black women in London, where one woman reported that the doctor was cross with her because she asked him to warm the speculum (Box, 1998).

Lack of privacy features only briefly as an explanation in the literature and where it does, the needs of the service are given preference above women's need for privacy. It is implicit in the requirement for male practitioners to have a female chaperone when taking the smear; and also in a study of the experiences of ethnic minority women (Naish et al., 1994), where most said that they found it too distracting to have children in the same room when having a smear test. However, there are no comparable findings of the presence of other health care workers in the room and the consequent lack of privacy. Lack of dignity is discussed in the literature mainly in relation to women's personal feelings of embarrassment. In both explanations of privacy and dignity, the focus appears to be upon the satisfactory taking of the smear rather than the circumstances surrounding the taking of the smear.

Surprisingly, the position of lying on an examination couch with her knees bent and legs open that women must (usually) take when undergoing a smear test has not been the subject of scrutiny within the literature, yet it appears to warrant discussion. McKie (1995) sets the smear test procedure within the context of the male right of physical access to women and the test mirrors the position frequently taken during heterosexual sex: these ideas are present in lesbians' explanations for disliking the 'missionary' position.

Experiences of smear tests

Painful experiences of smear tests

The most frequent explanation given by lesbians for considering that they had had an adverse experience of a cervical smear was 'Experiences of pain'. Lesbians commonly said that the test had caused pain; moreover, a number specifically stated that the health care worker contributed to the pain they experienced by their *clumsy, rough* or *brutal* handling. In their descriptions of their experiences, lesbians believed that health care workers underestimated the pain of the procedure: *I've only had two but on both occasions it was a bit of an ordeal. The medical types seem to think you can just shove things into a vagina & there is nobody attached to feel pain*. Others said that health care workers dismissed their concerns: *When the speculum was inserted it was very painful, I asked the GP to take it out and try again (as this sometimes happens during sex) but she said it couldn't be painful and just continued.* Yet others were silenced if the procedure was questioned: *felt inside me rough with her fingers. This I questioned at the time and was told it was practice.*

Among those experiences rated as good ones, painfree screening was the third most common explanation given. Lesbians said that there was *no discomfort from the procedure; the GP actually realize* [sic] *I had nerve endings; the experience was pain free; It didn't hurt and I didn't come out with my legs crossed!!* Lesbians spoke of *gentle* practitioners who *take great care to ensure comfort*. Other lesbians reported that their experience was in contrast to their expectations: *I was pleasantly surprised how comfortable I felt physically; I told her it had gone much better than I'd imagined possible.* These smears were taken with *integrity* and *care*.

Experiences of pain are usually associated with (presumed) heterosexual older women – who may find the test painful due to changes in the cervix; or socially anxious women – a woman's anxiety may prevent her from relaxing so that the test is needlessly painful. These findings appear to blame women themselves for experiencing pain during cervical screening. Furthermore, the recommended strategy has been to persuade women that having a smear test does not involve physical unpleasantness.

By contrast, others propose that the issue of pain rests with the skill of the health care worker: pain is due either to poor technique or to the health care worker not taking the time to help the woman to relax. Doctors sometimes underestimate the sensitivity of the cervix and women who have not had children are said to be particularly vulnerable. Tentative comparisons with findings in the mainstream literature suggest that lesbians' experiences of pain may be different; (presumed) heterosexual women are more likely to say that they found the test uncomfortable (44 per cent) than painful (10 per cent) (Schwartz et al., 1990). In the LHCS, lesbians were more likely to report pain (62 per cent) than they were to report discomfort (15 per cent). There were no comparable findings, which specifically attributed heterosexual women's experience of pain to the health care worker's lack of skill or care. However, in one study, young lesbians described how providers either went ahead with or stopped the pelvic exam and 'dismissed or ignored their articulations of discomfort or pain' (Scherzer, 2000: 95).

Among those who rated their experiences as good ones, practitioners were valued who acknowledged, rather than discounted, the possibility of pain. In relation to (presumed) heterosexual women, lesbians appear to be more likely to report painful experiences of smear tests. Those who reported pain-free experiences were most likely to attribute this to gentle practitioners who explained the procedure and took care to ensure their comfort at the time of the test.

Conclusion

In the mainstream literature, (presumed) heterosexual women rarely express dissatisfaction with even the most untoward health events; moreover, high-technology medicine – such as cervical screening – is viewed positively. In comparison with these findings, a substantial proportion of lesbians – 44 per cent – report adverse experiences of cervical screening. It seems that there are two possible conclusions to draw from these data. First, many studies that investigate women's evaluations of health care do so in the form of patient satisfaction surveys, which implicitly appear to presuppose a positive response; others are conducted in hospital settings where women may fear that their criticisms would get back to the staff concerned. By contrast, studies of lesbians' experiences of health care have often been conducted outside of clinical settings in the form of small-scale studies. It may be that the apparent differences between lesbian and heterosexual women's experiences of health care are in part due to different research settings and methodologies. The second possible conclusion is that lesbians are more likely to have had adverse experiences of health care than heterosexual women. This is not to suggest that if heterosexual women were asked about experiences of smear tests they would report only good ones. Clearly there are commonalities in both heterosexual and lesbian women's experiences of cervical screening: for example, they may be equally likely to report experiences of routine care or to report that the speculum was not warmed. But there also appear to be differences and these are exemplified in the three explanatory themes (i.e. experiences of pain or no pain; aspects of the procedure; attitudes and behaviour of health care workers). These themes will be considered in relation to improvements in health care delivery and strategies to promote equitable health care for lesbians.

Implementing lesbian-sensitive procedures

Cervical screening appears to be a more painful procedure for lesbians than for heterosexual women; it is the most frequent explanation given by lesbians for an adverse experience of a smear test. In comparison to findings about the experiences of (presumed) heterosexual women, lesbians were more likely to perceive that health care providers handled them in a rough, brutal or insensitive manner. Some lesbians said that the size of the speculum caused pain. Others said that the insertion of the speculum was a factor in their experience of pain. It may be that some lesbians do not engage in regular penetrative sexual activity and may experience the insertion or size of the speculum as particularly intrusive or painful. They may also anticipate intrusive questions: in two cases these were asked as the smear was being performed. If a heterosexual woman is asked about contraception or a partner after the insertion of the speculum, they are not faced with the decision about disclosure which may lead some lesbians to feel tense. Lesbians may also be apprehensive about coming out – some of them recounted heterosexist responses when they did disclose. Health care providers need to be aware of such differences and avoid blaming lesbians (as lesbians reported that they did) for finding the smear test an uncomfortable or painful procedure. In order to promote equitable health care for lesbians, health care workers need to be aware that some lesbians may be more likely to experience pain during cervical screening and to take practical (e.g. by the use of a smaller speculum) and attitudinal (e.g. by acknowledging that the procedure can be painful) steps to alleviate it. Furthermore, health care workers could respond positively to requests for a smaller size of speculum or routinely offer all women the choice of a range of size in specula and have these available so that they do not need to leave the room to get them.

Creating lesbian-positive environments

Strategies that health care workers can adopt to signal that the provision they offer is lesbian-positive can be done in a number of visible and immediate ways. Some health authorities have established 'equality in practice schemes' which provide training, resources and support to facilitate lesbians' access to primary care. In Leicester, the Lesbian, Gay and Bisexual Centre established Pink Triangle schemes in association with local GP surgeries. Some Community Health Councils have designed and printed leaflets that have addressed lesbians' concerns about cervical screening, while in New Zealand a health promotion campaign specifically targeted lesbians' need for smears. Health care settings can also demonstrate their active commitment to the nursing care of lesbians (and gay men) by displaying the RCN statement.

In addition, a range of practical measures can be implemented such as the use of appropriate language and terminology, and changes to patient registration forms and sexual history taking which allow either for lesbian self-disclosure or for the implicit acceptance of the diversity of women's sexual experiences and relationships. For example, the forms used by health care workers only allow for heterosexuality, as a participant illus-trated: *You've got to laugh, when I told the qualified nurse I don't use contracep-tives as I don't sleep with men her reply was 'Oh God there's not a box for that!' i.e. referring to the computer!* Others drew attention to the partial way in which their health care needs were met. They said that inappropriate questioning meant that they had to involuntarily come out or restricted what could be said. Lesbians as patients need assurance that their confi-dentiality will be maintained if they disclose their lesbianism. Moreover, if they choose not to have this information divulged in their patient notes such wishes should be respected. Being offered the choice of whether a female or male health care worker performs the smear test is more likely to contribute to a positive experience.

Developing anti-heterosexist attitudes and behaviour

Relationships with health professionals and the absence of heterosexism were key features in lesbians' positive evaluations of health care inter-actions. They were exemplified in the way questions were asked and assumptions were made (e.g. the lack of intrusive questions about con-traception or they were not assumed to be heterosexual). In some cases, lesbians reported that the atmosphere was generally supportive or the health care worker acknowledged their lesbianism. In other responses, lesbians saw the test as a chance to disclose their sexuality.

In their accounts of their screening experiences, lesbians said they were expected to counter heterosexist beliefs in health care interactions. Lesbians stated that they wanted information in a meaningful form from practitioners because they have spent some of their consultation time educating providers about their health care needs. Because of het-erosexism in the sexual health curricula, some participants said that their information needs about sexual practices were not met during the health care encounter:

> But they still didn't have much idea about lesbians. I had a possible genital wart and was concerned about safe sex to avoid passing it on as I had read of the communication between the wart virus and cervical cancer . . . when I explained why 'condom' wasn't appropriate they didn't have much idea what to say to me.

A principle of equitable health care for lesbians must be that there are not different expectations of lesbians as patients. One of the barriers to health care is the lack of information about the specific health needs of lesbians. Health professionals should be able to provide the same level of advice to lesbian as heterosexual patients about how they could avoid transmitting HPV to their partner. It was also very common for lesbians to report that they had received unequivocal advice from health care workers that they did not need a smear test, despite findings, elsewhere in the study, of positive smear results. Lesbian-sensitive providers should be aware that lesbian patients may expect rejection and prejudicial treatment and they may be more cautious than heterosexual women about disclosing personal information. Other examples of anti-heterosexist attitudes where staff placed value on lesbians' relationships included the recognition of a lesbian's support system or encouraging her partner to be present while the smear test was taken.

These issues have implications for the training and staff development of health care workers and they need to form an integral part of the nursing and medical curricula. Qualifying and in-service training can play a role in facilitating the provision of informed care: training has been shown to bring about positive attitude change and it can also provide a means for sharing good practice. Furthermore, creating systemic, institutional change will signal that lesbians are both recognised and valued as a patient group. The commitment to lesbians as service users has to be incorporated in institutional policies rather than be dependent upon the interest and commitment of individual members of staff. In addition, trade unions and professional bodies can follow the lead taken by the RCN and the RCM and include a comprehensive statement about the health care of lesbians.

Concluding comments

In contrast to the literature where adverse experiences seem to predominate, lesbians in the study were (slightly) more likely to report positive, rather than adverse, experiences of smear tests (46 per cent vs. 44 per cent). High levels of satisfaction have been noted elsewhere alongside accounts of disappointments and specific complaints (Wilton and Kaufmann, 2001). The findings suggest a positive basis for improvements in the delivery of cervical screening for lesbians. Good experiences were associated with the attitudes and behaviour of health professionals; by contrast, adverse experiences were more likely to be related to experiences of pain.

There are a number of limitations to this aspect of the study. First, it dichotomised positive and adverse experiences; many study participants took issue with this and suggested instead that their experiences were neutral. Others challenged the notion that there could be a good experience of cervical screening. For example, they said: *Can't imagine what would make it good?! It's like a trip to the dentist – not nice but it's got to be done.* Second, it did not ask whether participants had disclosed their sexual identity to the health professional performing the cervical smear. It may be that many lesbians in the study had not disclosed their sexual identity. Future studies which incorporate this question will be able to ascertain whether disclosure is related to positive or adverse experiences and whether disclosure increases the likelihood of lesbians' participation in cervical screening. Research which includes heterosexual women as a control group would be able to identify more clearly the similarities and differences between lesbian and heterosexual women's experiences.

8
Risky Bodies? Lesbians and Breast Cancer

Introducing risk

Risk is a central concept in understandings about health in western societies and its meaning has evolved over time. Previously, risk referred to probability; that is, it predicted the likelihood of an event occurring and this could have a negative or a positive outcome. In its current usage, risk is calculated by quantifying hazards and it has come to denote danger. In public health, risk is posed by two main factors: the environment, such as agricultural pesticides, which are external and outside the control of individuals; and lifestyle factors, such as smoking or lack of exercise, which are seen to be dependent on the choices made by individuals.

Risk is a biomedical term and is usually considered to be neutral in its application. In these approaches, risk is largely a rational weighing up of impartial technical information (Lupton, 1993). Some risk factors are highly associated with particular diseases, for example, high cholesterol with heart disease, smoking with lung cancer. They can be quantified; the risks posed by smoking are increased by the number of cigarettes smoked daily and the number of years an individual has smoked. Epidemiologists (researchers who study diseases) use risk factors to determine who is more susceptible to a disease and to identify the possible causes.

Biomedical approaches to risk

Breast cancer is a disease for which the cause is unknown. Because there is no one trigger, epidemiologists have identified instead a number of factors which make it more likely that particular groups of women will be at increased risk. Risk is not the same as cause; we know that in the case of cervical cancer up to 95 per cent of women have the human papilloma virus (HPV) and there is consensus that certain strains of HPV are the main cause of cervical cancer. When we compare cervical cancer risk to the risks of breast cancer, the risk story is quite different. This is because the known risk factors – including family history – account for less than 30 per cent of all breast cancers. Moreover, although women with family history are six times more likely to develop breast cancer than those without this risk, this means that women with no family history have a 1 in 30 risk, while women with family history have a 6 in 30 risk (Love, 1995).

Epidemiologists base their calculations of risk on large numbers of people. They observe a segment of the population – say 10 000 women – to see who develops the disease; they then estimate the relationship between the disease and the known characteristics of that population. When epidemiologists make decisions about risk (e.g. eating a high fat diet in the case of breast cancer), they compare the likelihood of the disease developing in groups of women with and without this risk. This is known as relative risk. While relative risk enables an individual woman to estimate her own chances of getting the disease, these calculations are not straightforward (Love, 1995). For example, risk factors do not increase like 'simple arithmetic': if one risk factor gives a woman a 20 per cent increase and a second gives a 10 per cent increase, it does not necessarily mean that a woman has a 30 per cent risk of the disease (Love, 1995: 182).

Risk factors for breast cancer include age, family history and environmental factors (e.g. pesticides). Because prevention is not possible (due to multiple risks), early detection is seen to be key in reducing mortality (the number of women dying) and morbidity (the number of women living with the disease). Women are thus encouraged to practise breast self-examination and to attend for routine breast screening when they reach the age of 50. The eligibility criterion is set at 50 because age is the biggest risk factor for the disease. In addition, a number of so-called lifestyle factors have been identified and they include a high fat diet, obesity, alcohol consumption, having children over the age of 30 and the combined contraceptive pill, alongside other factors which protect against breast cancer such as early childbirth and breastfeeding. Despite the appearance of neutrality, decisions about which risks to publicise (environmental vs. diet) are informed by mainstream attitudes and values.

Cultural constructions of risk groups

There has been an increasing emphasis in health education campaigns upon the risks posed by the lifestyle choices made by individuals because they are seen to be amenable to individual change. During the late 1980s, the concept of lifestyle risk was extended to groups, rather than merely individuals, said to be at increased risk of HIV. In characterising gay men as being at high risk of the disease, 'epidemiologists found themselves studying social behaviour embedded in values and beliefs – characteristics, which to the degree they are shared among and distinctive to a group of people, can be defined as culture' (Schiller et al., 1994: 1337). Gay men's risk of HIV was calculated on the questionable assumption that all gay men ascribe to a single set of cultural practices and values. In these discourses, risk is value-laden and based on assumptions that all gay men have multiple sexual partners and engage in specific sexual practices. The construction of gay men as a high risk group for HIV was informed by heterosexist beliefs that gay men as a group were socially deviant and by moral judgements that anal intercourse is less acceptable than heterosexual sex (which may include anal intercourse). An alternative approach may have been to inform the public, for example, that the probability of not contracting HIV in a single sexual encounter is 999 out of 1000; instead, 'focus [was] placed upon the one in 1000 probability that infection would occur' (Lupton, 1993: 433).

Lifestyle risk often emphasises responsibility and choice and takes on a gendered meaning in breast cancer discourse. It is the responsibility of an individual to avoid health risks; if they choose to ignore them, they are likely to place themselves in danger of contracting disease. As Yadlon (1997) points out, diet and reproduction are considered to be important risk factors and contain ideological assumptions about femininity. The culturally valued feminine body is slender and in order to attain this ideal, women must control their food intake. Reproduction is also associated with what it means to be a woman: having children is represented as the natural desire of women. Yadlon concludes by arguing that breast cancer discourse not only emerges from ideological assumptions but performs cultural work as well: the 'way to prevent the disease is to follow dominant codes of femininity' (1997: 647). These codes of femininity, however, are rooted in cultural constructions of a particular form of womanhood: heterosexual women. They are informed by ideological assumptions which privilege heterosexuality and do not represent the cultural practices of lesbians in quite the same way. Society does not expect lesbians to have children, and the little that is known about lesbians' cultural practices suggests that they might be more likely to resist heteronormative values embodied in a slender female form; moreover, lesbians' social history suggests that their socialising may involve meeting in places where alcohol is consumed. These competing understandings about women's roles and behaviours have led to the cultural construction of lesbians as deviant (or invisible) women in breast cancer risk discourses.

Media reporting of lesbians' breast cancer risk

The possibility of lesbians' increased risk for breast cancer became widely debated in the early 1990s following a study which suggested that some risk factors are more prevalent in lesbians. Suzanne Haynes' overview of these risks included: lesbians are less likely to have children; more likely to delay childbirth; more likely to drink alcohol; and are more likely to be overweight than heterosexual women. The ensuing media coverage sensationalised the findings by claims that 'One in three lesbians risks death from breast cancer' (Selvin, 1993) and 'The Other Epidemic: Lesbians and Breast Cancer' (Brownworth, 1993). The discussion was framed out of a 'rhetoric of panic' (Yadlon, 1997: 646). Many commentators have criticised the language of fear and danger, suggesting that lesbians have been singled out for media attention. Yet among (presumed) heterosexual women also, such representations are not uncommon: the disease is depicted as a particularly cruel cancer. The loss of life is said to be equivalent to a jumbo jet crashing every week of the year. Women are given the statistics of danger, but not the safety margins. Lupton (1993) argues that because the media is mainly interested in attracting a large readership, they tend to simplify information about health risks, but they also set the agenda for a public discussion of risks. The media reporting of breast cancer is probably one of the few occasions when lesbians' health has reached international attention.

There are, however, some important differences between the media reporting of breast cancer for heterosexual women and that of the coverage of lesbians. In reports of the disease in heterosexual women, the disease is a sexualised illness: it is young women's bodies and the sexiness of their breasts that makes breast cancer newsworthy (Saywell et al., 2000). Breasts are iconic of (heterosexual) women's sexuality and maternity and breast cancer in heterosexual women is seen as a violation of femininity. Heterosexual women are innocent victims of the disease. On the other hand, breast cancer among lesbians is seen to be caused by virtue of being lesbian. Socially undesirable characteristics such as obesity and heavy drinking are attributed to lesbians as a group; moreover, the risk factors confuse behaviour (e.g. having children) and identity (being lesbian). These differences are the basis of the lesbian breast cancer controversy.

What do we know about lesbians' breast cancer risk?

While sexual health and cervical cancer are among the most widely researched lesbian health risks, the increased attention to breast cancer has given impetus for a number of studies which have specifically targeted lesbians' breast cancer risk. There are two main areas which are the focus for study: risk factors and participation in screening.

In relation to risk factors, studies have investigated whether risk factors are more prevalent in lesbians. Taken together, they suggest that lesbians are more likely to drink heavily, less likely to have children, more likely to report breast biopsies and more likely to be overweight (Cochran et al., 2001). Lesbians, as individuals, may be no more likely to be overweight than heterosexual women; however, if 10 000 lesbians were compared to the same number of heterosexual women, lesbians may have a tendency to weigh more. Childlessness, not lesbianism, may be a risk factor for breast cancer. But if 28 per cent of lesbians have children compared to 67 per cent of heterosexual women, then among a large segment of the population, lesbians may be said to be more likely to be childfree (Cochran et al., 2001). Recent estimations by US epidemiologist, Susan Cochran, suggest there is not a lesbian breast cancer epidemic. Their increased risk relative to heterosexual women is considerably less than early calculations indicated. Lesbians have an increase of 11.1 per cent risk compared to 10.6 per cent risk among heterosexual women. The numbers mean that 110 000 out of 1 million lesbians would develop breast cancer compared to 106 000 of 1 million of their heterosexual sisters (retrieved 18 May 2005 from http://www.lesbianhealthinfo.org/events_news). These differences have implications for lesbians' breast cancer morbidity. A recent US population-based study lent support to the possibility that lesbians may be more likely to be living with the disease; it found higher prevalence rates of breast cancer among lesbians (Valanis et al., 2000).

In relation to screening, studies have shown that there are differences in breast health care between lesbians and heterosexual women: for instance, lesbians are less likely to practise breast self-examination and attend for mammography (Fish and Wilkinson, 2003a). If these findings are robust then lesbians would be at greater risk of dying from the disease because their breast lump was not detected sufficiently early. Although there is a growing body of research about lesbians and breast cancer, it will be some time before studies can establish lesbians' susceptibility for the disease or their mortality rates. There is, however, a common assumption among US lesbians that they are at increased risk for breast cancer (Solarz, 1999). Yet little is known about lesbians' risk perceptions because of lesbian invisibility within breast cancer discourses. In order to investigate perceptions of risk, the study collected quantitative data to ascertain how many participants believed that lesbians' risk is higher and qualitative data to explore the nature of their risk perceptions.

Combining data to explore risk perceptions

The study used a survey questionnaire which collected quantitative data through pre-categorised closed questions and qualitative data through the use of text boxes in which lesbians could provide discursive responses. In addition, the research methodology used a combined approach of focus groups – survey – focus groups. Although focus groups have been used previously in lesbian breast health research to inform the design of a survey questionnaire, they have not been used to explore survey findings. The rationale for using combined approaches was grounded in feminist research principles in which quantitative methods have the potential for transforming public opinion and qualitative methods enable consideration of perceptions of health and illness. Combined research methods are not commonly used to investigate risk perceptions:

> Research into the layperson's lifestyle risk tends to use quantitative methods, usually based on pen-and paper questionnaires that incorporate questions such as: How much risk (from the disease) do you think you are personally? with available responses ranging from 'at great risk' to 'not at all at risk'. Most questionnaires use only close-ended and pre-categorized items that provide very little opportunity for respondents to give unprompted opinions and to expand on their answers. These kinds of research methods into risk perception fail to take into account respondents' belief systems relating to causes of disease and health behaviours. (Lupton, 1993: 427).

By eliciting more detailed reasons for their attitudes and behaviour than is possible through traditional approaches, the study sought to explore lesbians' perceptions about health care and risk. Focus groups are useful for exploring the meaning of issues and concepts for particular groups of people while quantitative methods can generate the kind of really useful knowledge which feminist breast cancer campaigners need.

Quantitative data about risk perceptions

In the survey, lesbians were first asked to identify the main risk factors for breast cancer (for any woman). The question was open-ended and lesbians could identify as many – or as few – risks as they wished. In some responses, lesbians provided a list of what they believed to be the main risk factors; in others, they provided brief, but discursive, accounts of risk in which they reflected on what they knew and how that knowledge related to them as individuals: 901 lesbians responded to this question. By using content analysis, it is possible to count the number of lesbians who mentioned particular risks. This quantification provides an overview of the variety and diversity of their perceptions and gives an idea about the relative importance lesbians attach to different risks of breast cancer. Family history was the most common risk identified: 50 per cent (i.e. 454 lesbians, of 901) included this among the risks they described. These data are presented in Table 8.1.

Lesbians' perspectives on risk differ markedly from those posited in scientific explanations and perhaps reflect the amount of media attention devoted to hereditary risk. Family history accounts for between 5 and 10 per cent of women with breast cancer (Love, 1995); by contrast, 50 per cent of lesbians in the study believe that family history is a main risk factor. Furthermore, most breast cancer occurs in women over the age of 50 – about 80 per cent of cases; only 5 per cent of lesbians stated that age is a risk factor. Breast cancer in younger women attracts media attention and younger women with breast cancer tend to have a family history of the disease. Kylie Minogue, the Australian pop singer was recently feared to have breast cancer. Although the number of women under the age of 40 with breast cancer has increased by more than 50 per cent in a generation, the numbers are still quite small: in 1975, 14 in every 100 000 women under 40 were diagnosed with breast cancer. This figure rose to 22 by

Table 8.1:   Lesbians' perceptions of the main risk factors for breast cancer

Perceptions of breast cancer risk for all women	Number of responses	% of lesbians giving this response (N = 901)*
1. Family history	454	50
2. Smoking	349	38
3. High fat diet	160	18
4. Not having children	139	15
5. Death or danger	117	13
6. The pill	101	11
7. Not breast feeding	88	10
8. Don't know	77	9
9. Lack of early detection/screening	60	7
10. Alcohol	55	6
11. Age	43	5
12. Overweight	23	3
13. Other risks	599	66
Totals	2265	

*Figures do not add up to 100% because participants could give more than one reason.

2001. It is noteworthy that family history not only includes mothers (or other female family members) who had the disease pre-menopausally, but also fathers with prostate cancer; men with prostate cancer carry the same BRAC1 gene. Minogue's father had been diagnosed with prostate cancer.

Investigating lesbians' assessments of risk relative to heterosexual women

Lesbians were subsequently asked a pre-categorised item: *How do you see lesbians' risk of developing breast cancer?* The question allowed three alternative responses: *I think lesbians' risk is lower than straight women's.* The item was twice repeated for *same* and *higher*. This question aimed to investigate the widespread assumption among US lesbians that they are at higher risk of breast cancer. It has not been clear whether UK lesbians hold similar perceptions.

Of the 1014 participants who responded to this question (there were missing data from 52 participants); they overwhelmingly – 77 per cent – said that lesbians' risk is the same as heterosexual women's. Only 3 per cent said that lesbians' risk is lower; 18 per cent said lesbians' risk is higher and a further 2 per cent made multiple responses. These data are presented in Figure 8.1.

Because these quantitative data were surprising – in the light of assumptions of their higher risk – follow-up focus group discussions were conducted which enabled exploration of the ways in which points of view about risk are constructed and expressed. In the focus groups, because lesbians sometimes disagreed with each other, unexpected avenues were

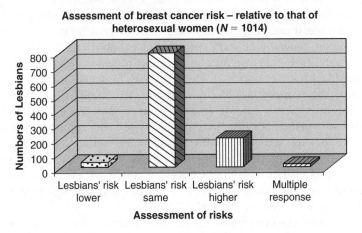

Figure 8.1: Lesbians' breast cancer risk relative to heterosexual women

explored. These qualitative data (both written and oral) offer insights that 'thick descriptions' can provide (Lupton et al., 1995: 90) about lesbians' understandings of breast cancer risk.

Qualitative data about risk perceptions

The following sections present data from the focus groups which explore lesbians' perceptions about the factors said to increase their risk of breast cancer, namely: (i) no children; (ii) drinking alcohol; (iii) being overweight; (iv) reduced participation in breast screening; and (v) risk perceptions in relation to heterosexual women. In each section, qualitative data are also presented from the survey, and where possible, they are followed by findings from other studies.

No children

Having children protects women against breast cancer and it is one of the biggest known factors in determining the overall risk. (It was listed fourth in lesbians' perceptions of breast cancer risk for all women.) Childless women are 50 per cent more likely to develop breast cancer than are women who have given birth. Moreover, women who delay their first pregnancy beyond the age of 30 are at significantly increased risk. For example, in comparison to women whose first child is born before they are 20, women aged 20–24 years at the birth of their first child have a 30 per cent risk, those aged 25–29 have a 60 per cent risk whereas those aged 30 or over (and those who have no biological children) have a 90 per cent risk (Rosenthal, 1997). Risk involves weighing up competing possibilities. While having children early offers protection for breast cancer, it also carries an increased risk for cervical cancer.

Women, generally, appear to be delaying childbirth until their careers are established. But there may be a number of reasons why lesbians are more likely to delay having children. Lesbians must take additional steps to plan their conceptions: deciding whether to conceive through formal or informal means, finding an appropriate donor and estimating the time of ovulation for insemination. Many lesbians appear to be older before they feel settled in relationships and are confident in their sexuality. Some suggest that doctors who provide donor insemination services use deliberate delaying tactics (including an extra counselling requirement and manipulation of the waiting list) to oblige lesbians to withdraw from services (Walker, 2001).

Breastfeeding – even for as little as three months – offers protection for pre-menopausal breast cancer. It was once believed that breastfeeding lowers the risk only for young women who breastfeed for long periods of time. Recent studies show that breastfeeding reduces the risks whatever the woman's age because lactation helps to eliminate carcinogens by secreting them through breast milk. Breastfeeding also appears to offer protection because it delays the return of the menstrual cycle after childbirth; hormones, produced by the lactating breast, may also provide protection. Although no research has been conducted about lesbians' breastfeeding behaviours, anecdotally it seems that they are as likely as heterosexual women to breastfeed their babies (Wilton, 2000).

In responding to a question about whether there was a shared perception of increased risk for breast cancer among lesbians, Kathy makes clear that it is childlessness and not lesbianism *per se* that increases the risk of breast cancer:

Kathy: I just heard that (. . .)
Maggie: Yes well it's been in the newspapers.
Kathy: Less in terms of lesbians than women who haven't had children (. . .) and what I'm suspicious of is: is that doctors saying 'go and get a child dear, you know you'll be all right'. Has that been an interpretation that's been put on the figures or are the figures really demonstrative that that's the risk?

Kathy problematises the notion of objective, value-free risk; she provides an illustration for the notion that if risk is socially constructed then we must consider the ways that scientific or medical institutions shape constructions of risk to achieve certain ends. Women are expected to have children. Kathy's scepticism highlights her concern that childlessness may be part of an ideological agenda, in which women who do not fulfil their 'natural' role as mothers and fail to conform to stereotypical notions of womanhood are deemed culpable for their increased breast cancer risk. In a subsequent focus group discussion, Dee provides an illustration of the way in which risk can be framed coercively. In this example, Dee's mother, who was unhappy about her being lesbian and childfree, used the risk of breast cancer as a means of persuading her to have children:

Dee: If you have breast fed, I believe you are at less risk of having breast cancer. Mum would say that to me you know. You haven't had any children and you might get breast cancer. And I'd say that's not a problem . . .
Debs: That's a bit of Welsh folklore.

While Dee acknowledges that she might be at increased risk because she has not breastfed, she also resists her mother's use of the threat of breast cancer to persuade her to have children. It is also interesting to note how a relatively established risk factor is reformulated, by her partner Debs, as folklore as a means of discounting the risk or perhaps to reassure Dee that the risk is not substantial.

In another discussion, Donna (a health professional) appears to suggest that breast cancer is more common in lesbians and that they have an increased number of risk factors. In her view, lesbians as a group have an increased risk of breast cancer, not only because they are less likely to have children than heterosexual women, but she also asserts that they are less likely to breastfeed:

Donna: (Breast cancer) it's more prevalent in lesbians for a start, because lesbians are *less* likely to have children – although I've got a three year old daughter myself – they're less likely to have breast fed. Erm so a number of things that do protect heterosexual women from breast cancer don't protect lesbians . . . but I think sort of lesbians are whammied on a lot of ways with breast diseases really.

As she talks about risk, Donna slips between talk about lesbians in general and herself in particular. Because she has had a child and has breastfed, she perceives her risk to be lower than lesbians as a group. However, in the following extract, she appears to recognise that, according to the opinion of medical professionals, she too has had her child late (which confers the same risk as having no children – she says it is the 'same thing') and is at possible increased risk for breast cancer:

Donna: I do think lesbians on the whole if they're in a lesbian relationship and choose to have children like I did erm they do tend to leave it till they're older anyway. I was 38 when I had my daughter erm and again late childbearing is the same thing (. . .) I breast fed my daughter for a year. I didn't really think about it at the time. Now I think erm this is really [inaudible] I thought I was quite clued up, well obviously, crikey.
Laura: What do you mean by late Donna?
Donna: Well over the age of 30 is classed as late by the medics.

Donna is obviously knowledgeable about breast cancer risk – she sees herself as 'clued up' – but the complexities of risk mean that multiple factors must be considered, rather than only one. In a focus group where none of the participants had children, lesbians enumerate the risk factors they know about and consider how they relate to lesbians. What is of interest to understanding how lesbians negotiate the complexity of breast cancer risk is that Robyn appears to try to offset the costs of having one risk with the benefits of not having another:

Robyn: Mainly we're . . .
Jo: Not having children.
Robyn: Not on the pill. We're not having the pill so it goes down, we're not having kids so it goes up.
Nikki: More and more lesbians are having children actually.
Jo: mm . . .
Robyn: What is the bigger risk though, is the bigger risk taking the pill or is the bigger risk not having a child?

Nikki challenges the assumption that lesbians do not have children. In the mid-1990s there were growing claims of a lesbian baby-boom both in academic articles and in the increasing media attention surrounding the birth of a daughter to lesbian rock star Melissa Etheridge and her then girl-friend Julie Cypher. A lesbian with children is not a recent phenomenon because many lesbians have had children from previous heterosexual rela-tionships. The notion of a lesbian baby-boom may reflect the growing tendency for lesbians, as a couple, to decide to have a child together.

Finally, in making their assessments of breast cancer risk, lesbians want to know whether the risk factor has been adequately researched:

Kirsten: What's the link between not having children? Is it well estab-lished?
Karen: mm . . .

The breast cancer controversy of the early 1990s has stifled research into lesbians' risk; consequently there is a dearth of information on which lesbians can base their assessments.

Lesbians in the survey, who responded to the question about *relative* risk, were more likely to cite no children than any other risk factor. Fifty-six per cent (N = 141, of 252) of explanations for lesbians' higher risk, stated that this was because lesbians were less likely to have children than heterosexual women. Many problematised the link rather than made a straightforward assertion that childlessness and lesbianism were associated. Some of these responses are presented below (the numbers relate to individual questionnaires which were allocated in the order they were received in the survey):

058   Less likely to have children – but that said lesbians who have had children are at lower risk than heterosexual women who haven't.

313   Depends on whether you have had children – I've read somewhere that there's a lower risk if you've had kids (true/false?) As a higher proportion of lesbians have not had children as compared to straight women, then I presume the risk is higher.

523   Probably slightly higher due to the factors around having children – i.e. lesbians probably tend to have them later in life or moreover choose not to have them at all.

535   Statistically we're less likely to have children.

Smaller numbers were aware of delayed childbearing as a risk and breastfeeding as a protective factor. In the focus groups, lesbians were both sceptical and in agreement with childlessness as a risk factor; they cited instances of risk being used coercively and they weighed their increased risk against other factors which afforded them protection.

Because reproduction is overwhelmingly associated with heterosexuality, the common assumption is that lesbians do not have children. This view was recently rehearsed as an argument against Civil Partnerships by a member of the House of Lords. In the US, it is thought that there are between 1 million and 5 million lesbian mothers.

Drinking alcohol

Drinking alcohol (some argue even in moderate amounts) increases the risk of breast cancer. Both alcohol and oestrogen are broken down in the liver and after many years of alcohol consumption, the liver is no longer able to metabolise oestrogen. The increase in levels of oestrogen in the blood is known to increase the risk of breast cancer in proportion to the amount of alcohol consumed. Women who usually drink between three and nine units weekly – the equivalent of nine small glasses of wine each week – have a 1.3 increase in relative risk, while those who have more than nine have a 1.6 increase (Love, 1995). The risk posed by alcohol consumption needs to be kept in perspective: if 1000 women over the age of 30 drank moderately for two years, one extra case of breast cancer might develop (Baum et al., 1994). The potential increased risk for breast cancer needs to be also balanced against the positive influence of moderate drinking on the heart.

Excess consumption of alcohol has long been associated with lesbians' lives. In a heterosexist climate, lesbians used alcohol as a means of reducing their social and psychological inhibitions. In her historical account of Fire Island, Esther Newton (1993) suggests that alcohol was the lifeblood of social occasions which revolved around cocktail parties, where alcohol was not only accepted, but conferred social status among middle class lesbians. Bars also provided important gathering places for working class lesbians when few other social venues were available to them. They were places where lesbians could occupy public spaces and make contact with other lesbians for friendship or romance. Bars were sufficiently clandestine to ensure privacy because it was not safe to be 'out' anywhere else; in them, lesbians could be themselves. Drinking in public places was largely the preserve of men; in the 1960s, drinking became a means for lesbians to challenge the prescriptions of femininity (Faderman, 1992). Moreover, bars encouraged drinking: there was pressure from bar staff for patrons to have a drink in front of them or leave.

In the focus groups, participants debated the place that bars occupied in lesbians' social lives and whether problem drinking was an issue. Kate suggests that lesbians drank because of the stress caused by hiding their sexual identity:

Kate: Maybe historically I don't know about now, I know that all the socialising 20 years ago was based around bars. That was probably more the pressures of not being able to be out for part of one's life or the whole of one's life (it) made for a lot of alcohol problems. But then it would be interesting (to know) whether younger dykes are also drinking as much I don't know.

Kate points to increased tolerance in the current social climate; there are now more social spaces for lesbians to meet each other. A quick glance through the community advertisements in *Diva* magazine reveals a host of social events for lesbians that do not rely on alcohol; groups for walking, sports, reading and drumming. The growing number of alternatives alongside increased tolerance may mean that lesbians have a greater range of choices for socialising and alcohol may become less of a feature of lesbians' social lives.

In the following extract, there is some dissension about the place of alcohol in lesbians' lives. Laura, Kate and Sonya present a range of reasons to explain lesbians' increased use of alcohol while Alison and Wendy present contrary evidence. In doing so, they show awareness of many of the debates surrounding lesbians and alcohol. Alison espouses the view, held by many current researchers, that by recruiting lesbians from bars, a distorted picture of their alcohol consumption is presented; Wendy draws on personal experience to support her case:

Laura: We do drink. To excess.
Kate: It's a cultural thing.
Laura: Gay, social, alcohol, bars.
Facilitator: You think we drink more than heterosexual women?
Laura: I remember seeing research that's from a few years ago now, three or four years, but I think it's the case that lesbians do use more alcohol.
Sonya: It's also the mundanity of the lesbians' lives that describes that culture of not being able to be out anywhere else so that's where you went . . . so you drank.
Alison: You see that research could have been flawed in the sense that erm the research, people who are researching were more likely to find lesbians who socialise in bars rather than the lesbians who weren't on the scene.
Kate: That would be true if it was research but I don't think it is. I think it's the cultural history of lesbians here and in the States probably, in that, you know, the only place they could go was to Gateways so that's where people went and because the pressure is on the rest of the week not to come out then it gets encoded.
Wendy: I've never sort of, I've never been a frequenter of bars anyway. I've never felt the need to be a frequenter of bars and I certainly don't drink a lot, my experience is that most of my friends don't drink a lot either.

Bars became the most important public manifestation of lesbian sub-culture and many researchers have used them as a means of recruiting lesbian participants to their studies (Lemp et al., 1995); however, many of the studies were about topics other than alcohol consumption, such as identities or HIV. Nevertheless, studies which did recruit participants from bars were likely to produce samples with characteristics that were atypical of the LGB population; bar users are often single, young, sexually active, drinkers and smokers. The studies referred to here about lesbians' drinking patterns did not recruit their samples from bars. It is not clear whether the tendency to sample from bars is a US phenomenon; there seem to be fewer examples in UK studies.

Not only have bars provided lesbians and gay men with a recognisable territory and community, but the bar has also been a site of cultural resistance. Bars hold a symbolic place in LGB culture because the Stonewall Inn – a New York bar – was the setting and catalyst for the launch of the Gay Liberation Front in June 1969 (when a group of lesbians and gay men fought back against repressive police tactics). Gay Pride marches have commemorated the Stonewall rebellion since the early 1970s in both the US and the UK (it has also given its name to a political lobbying and activist organisation in the UK). The Gateways bar (which Kate refers to above) has an emblematic place in lesbian social history because it was the setting for the first lesbian film, *The Killing of Sister George*, which, for many years, was the most commercially successful stage and film portrayal of lesbian relationships. The lesbian or gay bar, then, holds a place in LGB culture (notwithstanding its many limitations) because it is associated with political activism and visibility. Drinking is also cultural on other levels. At one time, a sign of being a 'real' lesbian rested upon the ability to drink only pints – rather than the half-pint measure typically associated with (heterosexual) women and emphasised by the euphemism: a ladies' glass. This notion of a culture of drinking is also referred to in the survey data. A range of explanations were offered to explain lesbians' increased likelihood of drinking more than heterosexual women including stress, lifestyle and opportunities for socialising:

208 And some of their lifestyle is largely [sic] based on high consumption of alcohol.

297 Lesbians drink slightly more, have more stressful lives in some ways.

362 From what I've seen, lesbians use alcohol and tobacco more prolifically than straight women.

1010 I suppose a higher number of younger lesbians socialise (smoke and drink more) for longer.

1055 Higher – because lesbians drink more – because of the need to frequent bars etc. . . . to meet other women.

Many people socialise around alcohol in their late teens and early twenties; one participant (1010) suggests that lesbians continue drinking for longer. Relatively few of the survey participants attributed lesbians' higher risk of breast cancer to their consumption of alcohol; however, they were twice as likely to say that lesbians smoked more than heterosexual women and thereby increase their risk. In response to a previous question about the main risk factors for breast cancer, 54 responses cited alcohol (see Table 8.1). This compares to 349 occasions where smoking was identified – even though the literature suggests that smoking is a non-risk factor for breast cancer. Baum et al. (1994) suggest that women who smoke have lower rates of breast cancer than non-smokers because of the anti-oestrogenic effect of smoking. However, there appears to be a widespread belief that smoking is a risk for breast cancer and there is anecdotal evidence that this assumption is shared by some doctors.

Studies of lesbians' use of alcohol have produced contradictory findings. Long-standing assumptions are that drinking does not decline (as it does in the population in general) as lesbians get older (Bergmark, 1999); lesbians are more likely to drink in bars and less likely to abstain from alcohol than heterosexual women (Ettorre, 2005); and younger lesbians drink heavily (Gruskin et al. 2001). Other studies have found limited support for the absence of a maturing out trend among lesbians (Parks and Hughes, 2005) and some studies suggest that there are no differences between lesbians' consumption of alcohol and that of heterosexual women (Hughes, 2003).

Being overweight as a risk factor for breast cancer

Being thin is synonymous with being beautiful and sexually attractive to men. The desire to be thin is so pervasive in western culture that up to 80 per cent of women wish to change their body shape or size by restricting their food intake: the ideal body size is declining among (presumed) heterosexual women. While the drive to thinness has led a number of heterosexual women to develop eating disorders and to be highly dissatisfied with their bodies, lesbians are said to be less concerned about conforming to stereotypical notions of femininity and are less subject to anorexia and bulimia. This is not to say that lesbians are immune to eating disorders or do not desire to be thin, but they are less likely to do so than heterosexual women.

Being overweight is currently constructed as a major health problem and rates of obesity are said to be rising. Women who have a higher body mass index (i.e. who are overweight) have a greater risk of post-menopausal breast cancer. Fat cells store and produce oestrogen thus increasing the risk of oestrogen-dependent cancers such as breast cancer. Women who are heavier than average (the 10 per cent in the heaviest group) have a 20 per cent increased risk above those women who are thinner than average (Rosenthal, 1997). Particular body shapes also increase the risk; women who have so-called apple shapes (women who carry their weight around their waist) are at higher risk than those with pear shapes (women who carry their weight around their hips, thighs and bottoms).

This is because fat around the waist is more metabolically active than fat carried elsewhere.

In both the survey and the focus groups, there were few data about weight as a risk factor among lesbians. Few women in the survey mentioned being overweight as a factor which might increase lesbians' risk; one participant drew on beliefs that lesbians rejected cultural expectations of thinness:

745   I think, in many ways lesbians are more likely to be 'overweight' – not so pressured by 'fashion' etc.

In the focus groups, some lesbians appeared to agree that being overweight may increase lesbians' risk. Others disputed the association:

Facilitator: Do you think obesity might affect lesbians differently?
Donna: I don't think so, (laughs) I think they are just as likely to be either slim or overweight as heterosexual women.

By and large, in the LHCS there was little discussion of weight as a risk factor for breast cancer. This may have been because they were unaware of 'being overweight' as a risk factor or that they did not believe that lesbians' weight differed from that of heterosexual women. The survey data appear to lend support for the first argument. When lesbians were asked *what do you think are the main risk factors for developing breast cancer?* there were only 23 instances of overweight as a risk factor (see Table 8.1). In comparison there were 454 instances of family history.

A number of studies have found that lesbians are at greater risk for overweight and obesity than heterosexual women (Cochran et al., 2001; Diamant and Wold, 2003). One study which used lesbians' heterosexual sisters as a control group found that while lesbians were the same height they weighed more than their heterosexual sisters (Rothblum and Factor, 2001). Furthermore, they were more likely to have the apple shaped body that increased the risk of breast cancer (Roberts et al., 2003).

Reduced participation in breast screening

Because breast cancer is a non-preventable disease, breast screening offers the best possibility for its early detection. There are three methods for screening for breast cancer: breast self-examination (BSE), clinical breast examination (CBE) (performed by a health professional) and mammography (an NHS service offered to all women aged 50 and above which uses X-rays to detect tumours). Because there are few studies which consider CBE among women generally, this section will explore breast self-examination and mammography.

Breast self-examination

Despite recent controversy in the UK surrounding the efficacy of BSE, biomedical sources continue to advise women to be familiar with their breasts and be aware of any changes; this is because as many as 90 per cent of breast lumps are found by women themselves. Lesbians are said to be less likely to practise breast self examination; in a comparison study, slightly more than twice the proportion of heterosexual women regularly practised BSE than did lesbians and lesbians delay seeking treatment for breast problems (Ellingson and Yarber, 1997). It may be that there is a higher risk of mortality among lesbians because their malignant lumps are not detected sufficiently early. Many lesbians do not practise BSE because they do not know what they are looking for, they do not know how to do it and they have never been shown (Fish and Wilkinson, 2003a). Heterosexual women are reminded to perform BSE when they attend for contraceptive advice or for smear tests; because lesbians are less likely to attend for these routine consultations they may be less likely to practise BSE regularly.

Personal instruction from a nurse or doctor increases the frequency of practice, particularly when a woman has been shown how to do BSE by one-to-one example (Fish and Wilkinson, 2003b). Being shown how to do it, is said to be the strongest influence for women to initiate BSE. In the focus groups, lesbians provided a range of experiences of health education around self-examination. In the first two extracts, lesbians themselves initiated the request and in both examples, they met with reluctance or hostility. In the third extract, Kerry describes being shown how to do BSE by the practice nurse who had initiated the advice:

Extract 1

Facilitator: What would help you to find out about how to do it (BSE)?

Faye: Erm yes, just show me physically. It's no good. I mean the last time I went for a smear test, she said you're OK. I said can you show me how to examine my breasts? And she said: like, well, we've got some pamphlets and she sort of pushes a handful at me and I was like fine then. That's fine, you don't want to show me because obviously I look dykey and I'm going to leap on top of you. You know what I mean: if you come anywhere near me. So I still don't know how to do it, I just physically don't know how to do it, so I don't. Pamphlets are no good.

Extract 2

Isabel: About two and half years ago I rang up the GP surgery and said I want to know how to examine my own breasts I felt like I should know. He said why do you want to do that. I said because I don't know. He was so funny with me . . . I went in and the nurse said to me so why did you want to know. I said I work in the health service and it's an area I don't feel very competent about and I should know how to do it. So she said well you just do it like this and she stood in the middle of the room and she moved her hand round her own breast and then she sat down again and she said there you go that's how you do it (laughs a little). So you just go like this and she said that's fine that's it and here's a little leaflet and off you go (patronisingly) (laughs). It wasn't very helpful. So I mean I do know, I obviously know now, how to self examine my own breast and through trial and error.

Extract 3

Facilitator: So how would you find out about doing breast self exam if you're not sure how to do it?
Kerry: Get a leaflet yes (laughs).
Nicola: I don't always believe in a leaflet, I think you should be (pause) shown properly (. . .)
Kerry: When she did my MOT I think she did vaguely explain to me how to do it.
Nicola: Did she explain or did she show you?
Kerry: I think she showed me actually. I seem to remember that she did do it at the time.
Facilitator: On her or you?
Kerry: Me, on me. And she told me off because I had not been for a smear test.

Faye's account suggests that the health care worker is reluctant to show her how to do BSE because she looks like a lesbian. Isabel has been particularly assertive in her request for BSE health education, having met resistance from both the GP and the practice nurse. The nurse, who does show her how to practise BSE, distances herself from Isabel by standing in the middle of the room. In both examples, the nurses seem to see the interaction as a potentially sexualised encounter. Other studies in lesbian health suggest that health care workers are reluctant to have any physical contact with lesbians (White and Dull, 1998); nowhere in the literature do heterosexual women report a similar reluctance by health care workers in relation to BSE. However, a study of heterosexual women's experiences of cervical screening found that participants' husbands viewed the smear test as a sexualised encounter in which male doctors took pleasure from performing smears and women themselves derived some form of sexual enjoyment (McKie, 1996). Moreover, one of the women in the study delayed going to see her GP about a breast lump because 'he always has the smirk on his face. I always feel that he's looking at my body' (McKie, 1996: 130). In the third extract above, Kerry reports being shown how to do BSE (although she has some difficulty recalling it) by the practice nurse, who takes the opportunity to remind her to have a smear test.

Breast screening (mammography)

A nationwide service of three-yearly mammography aged 50–64 was established in the UK and began inviting women for screening in 1991. The programme targets older women because they are at increased risk and because the technique (mammography) used for detecting breast lumps is unreliable in younger women as they have denser breast tissue. Women can ask their GP to refer them to a hospital breast clinic if they are concerned about a specific breast problem or otherwise worried about the risk of breast cancer (this is a diagnostic test). It is not part of the NHS Breast Screening Programme, which uses a routine call and recall system to invite well women. However, the same techniques are used in both breast screening clinics and hospital breast clinics for diagnosing breast cancer. Proponents of mammography claim that it is the only breast cancer screening method for which the value has been quantitatively demonstrated. The NHS Breast Screening Programme has screened more than 14 million women and has detected over 80 000 cancers: 300 women's lives a year have been saved. The success of mammography in reducing breast cancer mortality is reliant upon as many women as possible presenting for breast screening every three years from the age of 50.

Approximately 25 per cent of all women do not attend for breast screening and a number of studies have investigated why they fail to do so. In the mainstream literature, women's non-attendance has been largely attributed to so-called personal factors. Women do not attend for mammograms because they anticipate pain, they have misconceptions about mammography, they have a sense of fatalism or they prefer not to know they have cancer. Among ethnic minority women in the UK, there is assumed to be a causal relationship between information and uptake

(Chiu and Knight, 1999). Suggested measures for improving uptake include increasing awareness, addressing misconceptions and creating a health care environment conducive to the needs of the target population. There have been few studies which have investigated the reasons for lesbians' attendance or non-attendance, much less the nature of their screening experiences. In the focus groups, lesbians described their participation in breast screening:

Dee: I think mammograms are really important.
Debs: Well even the manual checks by the GP you know would be more useful. If they were done on a regular basis, rather than just abandoning you for three years. Stick your tits in a machine, go over there, that'll do, come back in three years.
Toni: Yes.
Debs: You know, that's how it feels, doesn't it? Get them in here that's it . . .
Carol: (laughs)
Debs: There's no, like, care about it, no . . .
Toni: No.
Becky: Well, when I had a mammogram I felt like I was at Kwik Fit.
Debs: Yes!

This extract develops our understanding of lesbians' experiences, because instead of merely reporting that she had been treated in a routine manner (as survey participants did), Debs offers what appears to be a representation of a typical mammography interaction. Explanations of the procedure are delivered as barked instructions – Stick your tits in a machine, go over there, that'll do, come back in three years – and it is evident that such poor communication is not conducive to effective health care. Debs' experience is clearly recognised by Becky, who is able to provide a metaphor for the intervention: she says it is like Kwik Fit (a car maintenance firm which advertises itself as speedy). This kind of hurried procedure is obviously not conducive to client satisfaction with health care provision. In another discussion, participants said that mammograms contributed to early detection:

Facilitator: Can I ask you whether you've ever had a mammogram?
Laura: I had that experience.
Sonya: Not pleasant.
Laura: No, very odd, I didn't mind at all (. . .)
Sonya: I've had two triggered early. It wasn't upsetting.

Laura: No, no it didn't hurt.
Sonya: Neutral is probably . . .
Laura: You do get squashed into funny shapes.
Sonya: You do get squashed a bit.
Laura: Pretty neutral though, I'd say.
Sonya: I'm happy to have it, have you feel (. . .)
Wendy: Anything that you can do that will help.
Sonya: Yes.

This discussion produces a neutral account of mammography. Sonya's initial assessment of 'not pleasant' is modified by Laura's perceptions of no pain. Although they arrive together at an assessment which depicts it as neutral, Wendy says mammography helps her to feel that she is looking after her own health.

In the survey, participants attributed lesbians' increased risk of breast cancer to their reduced access to screening and this was due to the anticipation of heterosexism from health care workers; the lack of knowledge of health care workers; and to the service (appearing to be) directed to the needs of heterosexual women:

329 There is fear of poor access to appropriate health care & fear of homophobia which keeps lesbians away from health care professionals.
488 Because they are less likely to get checked out – because of attitudes of health professionals.
535 If breast exams *do* help, then we're more likely to miss out if we don't go to clinics and doctors for contraception.
954 Because lesbians tend to feel excluded from mainstream medical services + would be less likely to seek attention.

There have been competing findings about lesbians' participation in breast screening programmes. Early studies suggested that lesbians received fewer mammograms; more recent studies have suggested that lesbians attend at similar or higher rates as heterosexual women. However, research conducted in the UK suggests that lesbians are less likely than heterosexual women to reattend (Fish and Anthony, 2005). There are important differences in health policy between the USA and the UK. In the USA, a baseline mammogram is offered to women from the age of 30 and they are offered breast screening annually from the age of 40. In the UK, heterosexual and lesbian women are not invited for mammography until they reach 50 (although there have been pilot studies for 40-year-olds). At the time the LHCS survey was conducted, the NHS programme only offered screening to the 50–64 age group.

Risk perceptions in relation to heterosexual women

The majority of lesbians perceived their risk of breast cancer to be the same as that of heterosexual women (see Fig. 8.1). In the qualitative survey data, there were two main arguments used to support participants' perceptions that lesbians' risk is the same and these are: being lesbian is not a risk factor for breast cancer; and breast cancer is a disease of women.

Being lesbian is not a risk factor for breast cancer

Many researchers who are critical about the suggestion that lesbians may be at increased risk for breast cancer, have expressed their concern that lesbianism *per se* may be seen as a risk factor. These concerns are understandable in the light of historical perspectives which have constructed lesbians' health as pathological (see Chapter 1). Wilton (2000) argues that the suggestion that lesbians are at higher risk for breast cancer – because of not having children, obesity and increased alcohol consumption – may collude with homophobic claims that lesbians are sick or abnormal.

But the failure to consider the possibility that lesbians, as a group, may have different risks has a number of important consequences. First, it contributes to heterosexist claims that lesbians are essentially the same as heterosexual women. Because there are no diseases unique to lesbians, biomedical perspectives appear to assume that lesbians have no distinctive health concerns: one of the biggest issues facing lesbians is the continuing invisibility of their health needs. While it is widely known that significant numbers of women develop breast cancer and many die from the disease, it is less well known that some of them are lesbians. Dibble and Roberts (2002) estimate that 12 210 lesbians were diagnosed with breast cancer and 2376 died from the disease in the US in 2002. Second, the possibility that research may be hijacked by those with conservative agendas and used to pathologise lesbians is not a reason for ignoring lesbians' breast cancer risk as there are other health concerns where lesbians may have worse health than heterosexual women (e.g. mental health or substance use). Third, it also ignores the social factors underlying lesbians' delay in having children (discussed above) or that for many lesbian and heterosexual women, being childfree is a positive choice. As Wilton (2000: 98) argues elsewhere, behaviours which do increase the risk of breast cancer are likely to play a different part in the lives of lesbian and non-lesbian women. If it were found, for example, that lesbians are more likely to drink heavily, we need to consider the social and psychological factors why this may be the case.

Participants in the survey said that being lesbian is not a risk factor for breast cancer. Many of the explanations simply asked why the risk should be different or alternatively a statement was made to this effect:

261 I can't see why risk of breast cancer should differ for the two groups.
275 I don't think sexual identity *per se* has anything to do with the risk factor.
395 I do not believe that sexual orientation has a particular bearing on the development of breast cancer.
691 Being lesbian *per se* has no bearing on the risks.
750 Lesbians come from all sections of the community, so I can't imagine why sexuality could be a risk factor.
1013 Being a lesbian or a hetero makes no difference.

In these explanations, lesbians assert that being lesbian is not related to risk. There are some parallels with the debates about 'risk groups' versus 'risk behaviour' which were extensively discussed during the early stages of the AIDS epidemic. The notion of risk groups characterised sections of the population (e.g. gay men, intravenous drug users) as engaging in culturally specific and exotic behaviours and stereotyped the behaviour of a sub-group as the norm for the whole group. For lesbians (and gay men), whose health has been traditionally pathologised in this way, there are many reasons to resist the categorisation of 'risk groups'. If lesbians were at higher risk, they would be deemed morally culpable for health risks which are attributable to voluntary factors. Lesbians' lifestyle choice to be childfree is used to apportion blame: their behaviour is the cause of their misfortune. Moreover, the question 'Are lesbians at different risk from heterosexual women?' is value laden. It cannot be read by lesbians as neutral because it is never posed as 'Are lesbian and heterosexual women the same or different from each other?' but rather, 'In what ways are lesbians the same or different from heterosexuals?' Heterosexuality is always the norm.

Breast cancer is a disease of women

Breasts are the most visible marker of being female: they are the 'crown jewels of femininity' (Yalom, 1997: 1). Even though more women die of lung cancer, and cervical cancer affects only women, it is breast cancer which is seen to be the quintessential women's disease:

> Breast cancer is one of the most important diseases of women, not only because it is both common and serious, but because, unlike

many other serious conditions, it is a major concern of women even when they do not have the disease. (Baum et al., 1994: 1)

Breast cancer is a major health problem among women in the UK, as it is for women in most Western countries. (Coney, 1995: 229)

While all cancers are frightening, breast cancer seems to hold the most terror for us as women. (Emmanuel et al., 1989: 535)

Breast cancer has been claimed as a feminist issue; feminists have exposed misogynist medical practices, such as the radical mastectomy and long referral waiting times. By redefining it as a women's health issue, breast cancer has become a 'kind of success story' for the women's health movement: in terms of raising the profile, campaigns for improving access to care and in fund-raising efforts among women to support research and treatment (Potts, 2000: 4). This redefinition has been part of wider campaigning efforts to change biomedical views and practice in relation to women's health issues: to distinguish their health needs from those of men and to recognise that health concerns traditionally seen as male, such as heart disease, are also concerns for women. But the process of making women visible in health matters has, of necessity, focused attention on shared experiences and on the similarities between women. For example, the key campaigning issue in the women's health movement has been uncompromised access to contraception and abortion; however, reproductive rights are not the same for all women. For black women, the issue is not to control their own fertility, but rather to resist unwanted birth control, forced sterilisations and abortions. For lesbians, reproductive rights means (among other things) equal and safe access to insemination services. The definition of reproductive rights as the core women's health issue clearly homogenised women's experiences and obscured the differences between them. Similarly, women do not have the same experiences of breast cancer: the incidence is lower among black women, but they are more likely to die from the disease; lesbians may also have different experiences of the disease. For example, Dibble and Roberts (2002) suggest that lesbians reported significantly more problems from chemotherapy-induced side-effects and were less satisfied with their physician's care than were heterosexual women.

Any discussion of different breast cancer risks seems to imply that breast cancer is a lesbian disease rather than a disease which affects both lesbian and heterosexual women. The hegemonic use of the word 'woman' to imply heterosexual women has erased lesbians' experiences from breast cancer debates, but the struggle to include them is taken, by some, as hijacking the breast cancer debate by lesbians. The emphasis on similarities and shared experiences (epitomised in the notion of sister-hood) has been a key principle of feminist campaigning and these discur-sive practices have shaped lesbians' perceptions of breast cancer.

In the qualitative survey data, lesbians frequently described their risk with reference to their similarity to heterosexual women. Their accounts drew upon feminist perspectives of breast cancer as a women's health issue. Being women gives both lesbians and heterosexual women the same risk of breast cancer. Some responses drew explicitly on biomedical beliefs that biology shapes women's experiences of illness. In their expla-nations, lesbians emphasised their similarity to heterosexual women on the basis of their shared biology: their bodies and their breasts. Hence lesbians' risk for the disease is the same:

160   Female bodies are the same irrespective of sexual preferences.
214   We are all women we all have breasts.
256   Breasts are breasts at the end of the day.
469   Every womens body is the same [sic].
1036   We are all built the same so we all have the same risks.

Being a woman is not usually identified as a risk factor for breast cancer in the scientific and popular literature (although for an exception see Love, 1995: 182, 'By virtue of being women, we are at risk for breast can-cer'). But breast cancer is not a women's disease in quite the same way as gynaecological cancers are women's diseases, because men can get breast cancer too. It is comparatively rare in men – only about 200 men a year develop the disease (approximately 1 per cent of cases) and it tends to occur at an older age.

Moreover, the suggestion that there may be differences between les-bians' and heterosexual women's risk of breast cancer appears to call into question lesbians' status as women. Lesbians have historically been considered to be biologically inferior to heterosexual women (see Chapter 1). Further, the female hormone oestrogen is implicated in breast cancer risk; lesbians have been considered to be hormonally masculine. Lesbians' responses are shaped by these assumptions and they make (either hesi-tant or assertive) claims to being women:

425   Women are women are women. Lesbians are women.
462   We are still women *aren't we* (emphasis added).

561   I'm still a woman – so I am at the same risk as a straight women.
843   Who we choose to have sex with doesn't take away the fact that we
        are women.
849   Lesbians are women!

Conclusion

This chapter provides one of the first investigations of lesbians' assessments and perceptions of breast cancer risk. Lesbians in the study do not
believe that their risk of breast cancer is higher than that of heterosexual
women: three-quarters of them stated that their risk is the same. In terms
of overall risk, family history is most often cited and they are much less
likely to know about other risks such as alcohol consumption and being
overweight. In terms of relative risk to heterosexual women, lesbians are
most likely to state not having children as a factor which may increase
their risk. Their accounts provide insight into the ways in which lesbians
talk about risk in the context of their lived experiences. They interrogate
scientific notions of risk as potential tools of ideological control in relation to having children. Although there is no consensus among them
about lesbians' likelihood of increased alcohol consumption, their explanations take account of social oppression. Many reject the suggestion that
their health risks may be different because they see this as an indicator of
pathology or as a challenge to their status as women.

The notion of risk draws upon biomedical discourses; as researchers and
activists we need to be wary of an over-reliance on medical models. One
definition suggested that 'a lesbian health issue was defined as diseases or
conditions which are unique, more prevalent, more serious and for which
risk factors and interventions are different in lesbians and sub-groups of
lesbians' (Plumb, 1997: 365). While the use of scientific discourse may be
a powerful means of persuading the medical establishment of the importance of lesbian health concerns, it may be inimical to lesbians' own
understandings of their health. It is not only important that lesbians have
knowledge about medical conceptions of breast cancer risk, but also that
epidemiologists and other researchers are aware of lesbians' constructions
of risk. Interpretive approaches which consider the relationship between
lay and expert knowledge of risk sometimes appear to privilege the latter.
Perhaps because of the methods used, lesbians' accounts of risk seem to
differ from those usually reported in research. Lay perspectives are often
characterised as fatalistic. Instead, lesbians weigh the costs and benefits of
risk; they balance scientific assessments with socio-political explanations
which take account of lesbian oppression.

Discursive practices have constructed lesbians' health as the same as that of heterosexual women (where lesbians' needs remain invisible and unaddressed) or as different from that of heterosexual women (where this is attributed to socially undesirable behaviour or pathology). Lesbians' breast cancer risk is, then, an example of the double bind of heterosexism. Same/ different dichotomous thinking about health needs is not unique to lesbians. Heterosexual feminists, campaigning for a separate agenda for women's health, faced similar challenges in their bid to differentiate (white heterosexual) women's health from that of men's: the male body and health problems had previously been the sole focus of concern. Health researchers are engaged in similar struggles to make lesbians' health visible by differentiating their health from that of heterosexual women. The challenge in this endeavour is to avoid reinscribing pathology.

9
New Directions in Equality Agendas: Opportunities and Threats

The legacies of political activism and lobbying

In their research into the changing politics of lesbian and gay equality in local government, Cooper et al. (2004) argue that there has been a marked shift away from conceptions of lesbian, gay and bisexual people as a class, which characterised early political movements. The political activism of the 1980s was successful in creating embryonic public spaces for lesbian, gay and bisexual people in community centres, help-lines, youth provision and support groups. Some local authorities adopted socially liberal and redistributive policies. The GLC gave financial support to emerging lesbian and gay groups: the newly opened LGB centre in London was the largest in Europe. The ensuing backlash in the form of section 28 and the accompanying cutbacks led to a retrenchment of services or served as a pretext for inaction for the most part of a decade from 1987–97. Lesbian and gay equality work was demonised by the tabloid press and local authorities were reluctant to support service provision out of fears of being labelled 'loony left'; moreover, many saw the work as an electoral liability (Cooper et al., 2004). The legacy of the 1980s on current initiatives has been mixed. In some local authorities, it provided a foundation on which to build subsequent work; while others, notably Kent County Council, retained the provisions of section 28 or otherwise demonstrated their reluctance to embrace equality by refusing to register Civil Partnerships. The result is a piecemeal and fragmentary approach to lesbian and gay equality work in both the public and voluntary sectors.

The tactics of the 1990s involved coalition-based politics. In the face of an obstructive and recalcitrant House of Lords, the government was obliged to resort to the little used Parliament Act in order to force through age of consent legislation. The current approach is cautious, low profile and seeks change incrementally. In the UK, legislative change has been made acceptable by trade-offs: the first attempt at repeal of section 28 was preceded by new guidelines affirming the status of the heterosexual family and opposite-sex relationships in sex and relationships education (SRE) for schools. The SRE guidance, which remains current policy, states that children 'should learn the significance of marriage and stable relationships as key building blocks of community and society'. When the repeal failed amid much controversy, there was a three-year period where section 28 coexisted with the SRE to create a particularly hostile policy environment for lesbians, gay men and bisexuals. A backlash followed President Clinton's US election pledge to lift the ban on lesbians, gay men and bisexuals in the military. The capitulation to the right-wing led to the formulation of the *Don't ask, Don't tell* policy: lesbians and gay men can serve in the armed forces as long as they keep their sexual identity private. Those who fail to do so are dismissed. A further example of LGB civil rights' gains being overturned was in the reactionary Defense of Marriage Act 1996 which states that marriage is a union between a man and a woman. It was introduced under President Clinton following the recognition of same-sex unions in Hawaii. President Bush subsequently invalidated over 4000 same-sex unions in the early twenty-first century.

Equal citizenship?

Equal rights arguments can appear to be useful in making a powerful case that lesbians and gay men merit equal treatment to heterosexuals; however, being treated equally usually means being treated the same. The equality argument fails to recognise relationships of subordination and domination; it ignores the differences between homosexuals and heterosexuals which exist because of structural oppression and treats them as if they occupy a level playing field.

Equality rights discourses confuse equality of opportunity with equality of outcome. Moreover, they set the terms on which the debate is held by obliging LGB people to use liberal arguments, which emphasise their similarity to heterosexuals, rather than highlighting the substantive differences between them. For example, the debate about the age of consent was won, not on the basis of liberty (a lower age of consent than 18), but on the case for an equal age of consent with heterosexuals (this was seen to embody equality) (Waites, 2003). Equality was achieved by characterising homosexuals as the same as heterosexuals: the reduction in the age of consent ignored real differences between them. Gay and heterosexual young men do not make equivalent decisions to engage in sexual behaviour: young heterosexuals are not told that their desire is a passing phase; they are not liable to be thrown out of the family home for engaging in heterosexual sex; and it is unlikely that parents would blame themselves for their son's heterosexuality. By treating them as if they are the same, heterosexual young men are privileged. Many of the gains achieved at the turn of the twenty-first century have been liberal, individualised rights in the personal and domestic arena: adoption; age of consent; domestic violence; tenancy succession; immigration rights; gender recognition; and Civil Partnerships. This is not to deny the transformative potential of some of these civil rights on heterosexuality's key institutions, nor to suggest that they do not bring real benefits in the daily lives of LGB people. But they may make wider social change more problematic because they confer the appearance of equality. It is in the public domain where battles for equality are more difficult to accomplish because they rely on root and branch reform of the whole system; these are not just in structural and institutional systems which privilege heterosexuality, but also in the value bases and cultural practices which sustain those institutions.

Diversity and social inclusion

The language of current government policy initiatives emphasises diversity and social inclusion. The benefits of a diversity agenda are in the recognition of multiple identities; because of its inclusive focus, it may prevent heterosexual workers from distancing themselves from sexual minorities (Cooper et al., 2004). But it also appears to dilute the politics of the policy agenda. A parallel tendency towards inclusivity has been noted in public health research. There, inclusivity has been signalled in the use of the purportedly neutral term of 'men who have sex with men' (MSM) and the corresponding term for women (Young and Meyer, 2005). While the terms forced a conceptual shift towards the inclusion of diverse identities, including those without a sexual minority identity – such as married men – their usage has deflected attention away from the social dimensions of sexual identity. While MSM may avoid assumptions about a singular gay identity, its use may inadvertently lead to the erasure of political organising and LGB identities (Young and Meyer, 2005). As noted in the public sector report *Directions in Diversity*, unless they are specifically mentioned, LGB people can feel that so-called inclusive policies do not include them (Audit Commission, 2002).

The diversity agenda is not about treating everybody in the same way, but its starting point is the acknowledgement that inequity and discrimination exist in public services (Audit Commission, 2002). The report argues that the concept of diversity is complex and, because it has implications for policy and practice, there need to be shared definitions which form the criteria for measuring outcomes. However, evidence on the effectiveness of diversity strategies has thus far been scarce (Audit Commission, 2002). Improving access to services relies on monitoring systems that are non-existent for LGBT people. An organisation cannot tell whether its service user profile is representative of LGBT communities, because there are no government recognised data sets. These are needed if the historic invisibility of LGBT people as users of public services is to be addressed. In most public sector organisations, there has been no monitoring of LGBT people within the workforce at recruitment or at different grades within the organisation. The success of the diversity agenda, however, appears to rely heavily upon acceptance by public and private sector organisations of the business case for diversity. An example given in the *Directions in Diversity* report is that of a company's employee base being widened by recruitment among lesbian and gay graduates to a multinational financial organisation. Diversity in this formulation appears to rely on capitalism to end discrimination and oppression and is likely to benefit those LGBs who are most privileged: white, middle class and educated.

The CEHR: the new single equality body

It is against this backdrop that the government launched its most significant review of equality institutions in 2003. For a quarter of a century, the UK's equality institutions have been single strand: that is, a statutory body has been dedicated to each of the equality strands of: gender, 'race' and, more recently, disability. These are, respectively, the Equal Opportunities Commission (EOC), the Commission for Racial Equality (CRE) and the Disability Rights Commission (DRC). Yet, despite the introduction of anti-discrimination legislation thirty years ago – the Sex Discrimination Act 1975, the Race Discrimination Act 1976, and more recently, the Disability Discrimination Act 1995 – inequalities persist in relation to gender, race and disability. The government White Paper, *Fairness For All 2004*, signalled new directions in the thinking and approaches in the equalities agenda. A single statutory body, the Commission for Equality and Human Rights (CEHR), will take over the responsibilities of the existing commissions in 2008 and assume powers and duties for the promotion, enforcement and delivery of equality, human rights and good relations between communities. The vision for the new body is to promote a common culture of shared values that underpin citizenship and embed an ethos of human rights in workplaces, public services and communities in the UK.

The CEHR will be responsible, not only for the three existing equality strands, but also three strands not previously protected by statutory framework: sexual identity, age, religion and belief. Recent research suggests that those who are prejudiced against black people are twice as likely to be prejudiced against lesbians and gay men (Valentine and McDonald, 2004). Many argue, in the light of evidence of multiple prejudice, that the CEHR will be better placed to respond to cross-cutting agendas. The innovatory approach implied in the recognition of the existence of multiple identities allows for the possibility that people do not experience their identities separately. There are also many shared agendas: for example, black women, in particular Bangladeshi and Pakistani women, are more likely to live in poverty than other women. The potential presented by combining the responsibilities may mean that the new Commission is more effective in tackling multiple discrimination.

The proposals have, by and large, received a positive reception, despite initial concerns that some of the existing powers of the established commissions would be eroded and despite fears that the work could be diluted because of the wider remit (retrieved 9 November 2005 from http://www.fawcettsociety.org.uk/documents/Fawcett%20response%20to%20CEHR%20white%20paper(1).pdf). Each of the equality strands has been concerned that its issue is the least recognised and will have most difficulty in commanding adequate resources and attention when commissioners have competing priorities. Furthermore, research has suggested that sexual identity issues are rarely considered to be of sufficient importance to merit a place on decision-making agendas (Cooper et al., 2004). The merger of the different equality strands might also imply homogeneity in the experience of discrimination and in the mechanisms for tackling it. For example, the heterosexism experienced by a black lesbian is different to that experienced by a white lesbian (see Chapter 3). The CEHR will need to understand the complex ways in which identities and discrimination intersect. It will also need to determine which of its activities might be single strand and which might be cross strand. Previous initiatives, such as Safer Cities, have addressed issues where there has been a perception that they are located solely in some communities; subsequent attempts to add in consideration of sexual minorities led to less than effective outcomes (retrieved 9 November 2005 from http://www.stonewall.org.uk/documents/stonewall_fairness_for_all_response.doc). There are other aspects of equality agendas which may be particular to certain strands, for instance, pensions for older people (although this may disproportionately impact on women), equal pay for women, stop and search for black people.

Human rights

The new Commission will also have the responsibility for building a culture of respect for human rights. By contrast to equalities legislation, human rights were only recently incorporated into domestic statute by the Human Rights Act 1998 which came into effect in October 2000. The legislation has not succeeded in mainstreaming human rights into the practice of public bodies. Moreover, the lack of a public body with a promotional and educational role has left a gap between human rights litigation in the courts and public awareness about what human rights entail (retrieved 9 November 2005 from http://www.liberty-human-rights.org.uk/). The inclusion of human rights brings a new dimension to the equalities agenda, because they are based on the principles of fairness for everyone, not just those groups who experience discrimination. Some are concerned that the addition of a human rights agenda will bring a different focus; human rights' decisions are often made by balancing the rights of an individual against those of wider society. Human rights are sometimes perceived as conflicting with the rights of others, for instance, where the rights to privacy under the Data Protection Act 1998 conflict with a child's right to be protected enshrined in the Children Act 2004. Liberty has suggested that there is a perception that the HRA 1998 is a tool for criminals: Ian Huntley was able to gain employment as a school caretaker because evidence of his unsuitability to work near children was destroyed by Humberside police under mistaken assumptions about the provisions of the Data Protection Act 1998. Furthermore, some are concerned that the narrow focus of individualised rights makes it difficult to argue for wider social change (Rahman, 2004). Human rights are in danger of becoming the new hegemony and do not offer an immediate solution to the range of lesbian and gay inequalities. For example, the UK Parliament refused to include specific reference to sexual minorities in article 14 of the Human Rights Act 1998, which prohibits discrimination on grounds of 'race', gender and religion; it also failed to mention disability and age. But the inclusion of human rights may offer the potential for more co-ordinated strategies for tackling inequalities in public services: in addressing discrimination in health care, bullying in schools, and the delivery of residential care to the elderly. Human rights allow focus on public bodies not only as employers, but also as service providers; it also includes the private and voluntary sectors. As with the equality agenda, some aspects of the human rights have different relevance for each of the strands. Sarah Spencer (retrieved 9 November 2005 from http://www.ippr.org.uk). exemplifies this in her submission to the Joint Committee on Human Rights: privacy may be a prime concern for disabled people and older people. The right to family life is not a prime concern for most religious minorities, but it is for lesbians and gay men, for black people trying to secure family union through the immigration system, and older people in residential accommodation.

Existing and proposed equalities legislation

The Commission will bring together three long-standing areas of work (alongside three new ones); because of this history of a separate development there is a complex body of existing legislation. There are 39 Acts of Parliament, 38 statutory instruments, 12 European Community directives and 11 codes of practice in anti-discrimination legislation. The legislation identifies key measures on which discrimination occurs: direct discrimination; indirect discrimination; victimisation; harassment and bullying. At times, the legislation involves different definitions and interpretations of, for example, indirect discrimination. The scope of the legislation for gender, race and disability includes: education; housing; goods; facilities and services (public/private). The following section presents a brief consideration of existing and proposed legislation.

Gender

The Sex Discrimination Act 1975 prohibits discrimination in relation to employment, education, housing and the provision of goods and services. The Equal Pay Act 1970 was introduced to eliminate pay discrimination and other terms and conditions between men and women doing equivalent work.

The government is legislating for a public duty to promote gender equality by April 2007. There is governmental support for gender equality in the form of the women and equality unit and a minister with responsibility for women.

'Race'

The Race Relations Act 1976 prohibits discrimination in relation to employment, education, housing and the provision of goods, facilities and services and in the exercise of other public functions.

The Race Relations Amendment Act 2000 introduced a general statutory duty (sometimes called a public or a positive duty) to eliminate unlawful discrimination on the grounds of 'race', to promote race equality and good relations between communities. Public bodies must take account of racial equality in the everyday work of policy-making, service delivery, employment and other functions. It was partly introduced to combat the institutional racism highlighted by the Macpherson Report into the death of Stephen Lawrence.

Disability

The Disability Discrimination Act 1995 prohibits discrimination against disabled people. The Act is unique in equalities law in that it contains no equivalent prohibition in relation to those who are not disabled. The DDA (1995) creates a duty to make reasonable adjustments and prohibits discrimination in relation to employment, education, the provision of goods and services, and to a limited extent public transport.

The Disability Discrimination Bill 2005 proposes to introduce a general duty on public bodies to end unlawful discrimination and promote disability equality. The bill will extend the scope of disability to include more people with HIV, cancer and multiple sclerosis. It will also include measures for rail accessibility.

Religion or belief

The Employment Equality (Religion or Belief) Regulations 2003 prohibit direct and indirect discrimination and harassment on the grounds of religion or belief in employment and vocational training. The legislation includes discrimination on the grounds that a person has no particular religion or belief.

Sexual orientation

The Employment Equality (Sexual Orientation) Regulations 2003 prohibit direct and indirect discrimination and harassment on grounds of sexual orientation in the fields of employment and vocational training.

Age

The EC Employment Directive requires EU member states to prohibit age discrimination. The proposed regulations will be introduced by December 2006 and will prohibit direct and indirect discrimination and harassment on the grounds of age in the fields of employment and vocational training.

Among the submissions to the consultation phase, LGBT groups and communities largely saw the establishment of the new Commission as positive because previously, there was no regulatory body to promote or protect the rights of LGB. Their support needs to be understood within this context and within the differential policy and legal framework. Any discussion of the disparities between equality strands needs to balance acknowledgement of the importance of human rights and equality legislation in meeting the needs of disadvantaged groups with the recognition of the differences between them. In presenting the following analysis, the intention is not to claim that LGBT people experience greater oppression than other groups, but rather to point to the anomalies and the barriers to their claims to equal citizenship.

Hierarchy of equalities

There appears to be an inconsistency between the government's vision of a fairer society for all and the differences in the scope of the legislation that underpins this commitment. Significantly, the government has refused to implement a single equality framework, which would harmonise existing equality legislation, citing concerns from private sector respondents that this would distract the CEHR from the important task of bedding down new areas of employment discrimination law (retrieved 6 November 2005 from http://www.dti.gov.uk/consultations/files/publication-1407.pdf). Some of the key differences are discussed below.

Although the EER (2003) did not extend to discrimination in the provision of goods and services for religion and belief, age and sexual identity, the government is proposing to extend protection in the provision of goods, facilities, services and premises on the grounds of religion and belief in new legislation (retrieved 6 November 2005 from http://www.dti.gov.uk/consultations/files/publication-1407.pdf). It is also actively considering extension to public functions.

The government has included transsexual and transgender people in the CEHR's duties to promote good relations between different communities. It has not, however, assigned specific responsibilities under the Gender Recognition Act 2003. Transgender people are protected against discrimination in the provision of education and vocational training. They are not protected from discrimination in the provision of goods and services.

The White Paper laid out provisions for a statutory requirement for a disabled Commissioner and for the establishment of a disability committee with at least 50 per cent disabled members. The vision for the single equality body did not envisage the appointment of Commissioners as champions of particular equality strands and did not allow for the appointment of other Commissioners with the lived experience of inequalities. The CEHR will have the power to establish committees with delegated functions, for example, on race equality. However, the Commissioner for public appointments has not been asked to ensure the representation of LGB people on public bodies (retrieved 9 November 2005 from http://www.stonewall.org.uk/documents/stonewall_fairness_for_all_response.doc). The lived experience of sexual identity does not appear to be valued by government ministers.

Discrimination in education on the grounds of sexual identity will not be prohibited by the EER (SO) (2003). The government may reconsider its initial refusal to extend protection to lesbians, gay men, bisexuals and transgender people in the delivery of goods, services and facilities following a proposed new clause by Lord Ali (retrieved 9 November 2005 from http://www.cre.org.uk).

There is no commitment to introduce a public duty for sexual identity equality.

The case for a positive duty on sexual identity

The introduction of a public duty presents important opportunities for mainstreaming race, disability and gender into public services. The new duty requires public bodies – e.g. the police, health services, education, local authorities, and social services – to eliminate unlawful discrimination and promote equality. It offers the potential for tackling structural inequalities, rather than merely providing redress once discrimination has occurred. The legislation injects the concept of mainstreaming equalities into the decision-making of public sector bodies both in relation to the services provided and their internal employment policies. The term 'mainstreaming' refers to the normative assumptions, attitudes and activities of society and is achieved by incorporating a 'race', disability and gender perspective into all policies and programmes. Mainstreaming, then, is a strategy for achieving equality, alongside existing equality policies. In relation to employment practices, public bodies will be required to monitor the composition of their workforces and applicants for jobs, promotions and training by 'race', disability and gender. Larger authorities will be obliged to monitor grievances, disciplinary action, performance appraisals, dismissals and training. In relation to services, public bodies will be required to understand the implications of their policies for equality strands leading to a better user focus in policy development and practice guidelines. Specifically, public bodies will need to (i) assess whether their functions and policies are relevant to 'race', disability and gender equality; (ii) monitor their policies to consider how they affect equality; (iii) publish results of the monitoring, assessments and consultations;

(iv) ensure public access to information; (v) provide training for staff on new duties.

A positive duty for sexual identity would require public bodies to take account of the needs of LGBT people in the design and implementation of services and employment practices. A sexual identity mainstreaming strategy introduces a sexual identity perspective (known as impact assessments) into a particular policy field and helps policy-makers explore how policy objectives affect different sections of the community, how services are accessed and whether policies are delivering results for the intended user group. But the question remains for policy-makers: what are the barriers to producing a sexual identity mainstreaming strategy? The Women and Equality Unit provide a framework of activities (retrieved 9 January 2003 from http://www.womens-unit.gov.uk/gender_mainstreaming/explanation.htm) for a gender mainstreaming strategy and this is used to explore the barriers to producing a sexual identity mainstreaming strategy. It includes sponsorship, awareness raising, training on equality issues, equalities expertise, research, statistics and resources.

Sponsorship

The strategy proposes a sponsor who will drive the mainstreaming strategy, allocate resources, develop knowledge of equality strand issues and implement policies containing equality strand perspectives. Sponsorship of LGBT equality initiatives has been distributed across government departments, such as the WEU for Civil Partnerships, the DTI for Equality Employment Regulations, DFES for homophobic bullying in schools and the DH initiated external reference group on sexual orientation. The result of this has been a piecemeal approach which has dissipated expertise. To date, there are few policies containing a sexual identity perspective.

Awareness raising

Although in relation to gender, individual policy-makers will not necessarily have knowledge of social structures and gendered patterns of behaviour, there is well-developed body of theory and practice to support this understanding. This is not generally the case for sexual identity where concepts for understanding heterosexism, how it impacts the delivery of services and the ways that institutions are organised are less developed. More work needs to be done, for example, to understand the specificity of lesbians' experiences of public services – what is lesbian about lesbians' experiences of health service provision? We need to develop understanding of such concepts as institutional heterosexism, indirect discrimination and harassment. An anti-oppressive approach which affirms LGBT identities is needed to link the personal with the political where an individual's life situation is understood in the context of heterosexist social systems, together with recognition of disparities in power and social difference. We need to understand the cultural, economic, psychological, social and structural impacts of heterosexism, in its historical context and in different geographical locations. We need to be mindful of the ways that those with intersecting identities experience heterosexism and how dominant values can be challenged.

Training on sexual identity issues

The strategy advises the use of specialists in academic and voluntary sectors and emphasises the on-going nature of the work. There is a tradition of lesbian and gay awareness training in public and private sector organisations, but its implementation has not been as systematic as that for gender. Consequently, the range of materials to support such training may be less developed.

Sexual identity expertise

In comparison to 'race', disability and gender, where a number of long-established organisations have been active in the not for profit sector, one of the legacies of section 28 has meant that there is little LGBT community infrastructure. This is partly evidenced by the number of organisations responding by equality strand to the *Fairness For All* consultation document. The LGBT voluntary sector largely exists on short-term grants from a number of different bodies; the lack of consistent funding results in a major focus on fund-raising and balancing competing priorities. This may have resulted in the reduction in the number of experts in the voluntary sector, central and local government and in academic institutions.

Research

Policy-making which is sensitive to sexual identity differences and the provision of services tailored to meet their needs is dependent upon valid and reliable research. Existing research does not provide national information across the breadth and depth of policy areas for sexual minorities. Without data on the characteristics, circumstances and needs of LGBT communities, there is a lack of clarity about policy priorities and the delivery of services. Even in Scotland – where, since devolution, the Scottish Executive and NHS Scotland have taken a lead in commissioning research – there is a need for greater harmonisation. The lack of a centralised approach has also led to some duplication of research efforts and poor dissemination of findings. Despite efforts by voluntary groups to make research accessible, there is no central point of contact for community organisations, service providers, funders and policy-makers (McLean and O'Connor, 2003).

Chapter 4 identified some of the reasons for these gaps in the research base. Chapter 2 attempted to address these gaps by providing an overview of current UK research in LGB health and social care needs. In Brighton, the city with the proportionately largest LGB population in the UK, local activists and researchers conducted a needs assessment and developed a comprehensive strategy to address priorities, yet none of the major public bodies has responded strategically to the needs highlighted (Count me in, retrieved 5 May 2005 from http://www.spectrum.org.uk). Some argue that 'irrefutable evidence or proof' is needed, in the form of robust enquiries, for agencies to respond (McLean and O'Connor, 2003: 2), yet without adequate funding, LGBT research remains trapped in a Catch-22 situation. As Plumb (2001) argues, without funding we cannot do quality research, and without quality research we cannot convince that a need exists.

Statistics

In order for a mainstreaming strategy to be effective, there needs to be relevant data available to inform, monitor and evaluate progress made towards equality goals. For example, the CRE is able to draw on data analysed by ethnic group in relation to the population as a whole (although there are limitations) and also to particular policy areas including health, housing, criminal justice, education and the labour market. Surveys have collected data over a number of years so that it is possible to analyse trends, for example, in access to health care. There are no statistics in relation to sexual minorities. This means that the White Paper was unable to provide a coherent rationale for responding to new challenges for LGBT people; because, in contrast to each of the other equality strands, it does not have access to basic information about the size of the LGBT population in the UK (retrieved 9 November 2005 from http://www.dti.gov.uk). Although the census included an item on sexual identity for the first time in 2001, efforts need to be made to recognise them as an under-enumerated group and to facilitate disclosure (retrieved 14 December 2005 from http://www.statistics.gov.uk).

In the USA, progress has been made towards the inclusion of LGBT issues in population-based studies and within the health policy agenda (Meyer, 2001). Importantly, by recognising inequalities in LGB health, the US government must establish systems to monitor services in order to ensure its objectives are achieved. Unlike the UK, half of the US

Department of Health and Human Services information systems have measured some aspect of sexual identity. In the UK this is a more challenging task because, for example, no systems have been established through the Public Health Laboratory Service Communicable Disease Surveillance Centre to collect data on STIs among lesbians.

Resources

Many of the building blocks are in place for developing and delivering mainstreaming strategies for other equality strands; for example, government departments have already incorporated a gender perspective into their policies. The techniques and tools for sexual identity mainstreaming are not well developed. There are relatively few mechanisms for engaging with stakeholders, such as contact databases and directories, working groups, round tables and conferences. Nor is there an established infrastructure of checklists, guidelines and impact assessment methods; however, some ground-breaking work has been conducted in relation to homophobic bullying in schools.

Conclusion

Devolution has had a positive impact for the health of LGBT in Scotland where the NHS has taken a lead in commissioning research and instituting an agenda for change. The initiative has led to an audit of current provision of LGBT targeted services, the establishment of demonstration projects and the sharing of innovative practice. Without a co-ordinated and systematic approach, health and social care equity cannot be achieved for LGBT people in the UK.

There is increasing evidence of change in our social institutions and cultural practices where a number of organisations have made important commitments to eradicating heterosexism and towards the social inclusion of LGBT people. But this shift must not be at the superficial level of tolerance and token change, but permeate the fabric of society and our attitudes towards sexual difference. A major issue for debate is how far recent developments, such as Civil Partnerships, mean that LGB people are becoming more like heterosexuals because of the security, recognition, financial and social benefits conferred through the new status or to what extent the institutions of society, such as marriage, are fundamentally changed by LGBT inclusion. The challenge is to change societal institutions, rather than become assimilated into heteronormative values and ways of thinking.

Appendices

Appendix A

Overview of historical and recent legislation

1885 The Labouchere Amendment

This created the offence of gross indecency and made all sexual acts between men illegal. It became known as the 'blackmailer's' charter. Oscar Wilde was prosecuted under this legislation. Until 1861, sex between men was punishable by death.

1967 Sexual Offences Act

Decriminalised homosexuality between two consenting men, in private, providing both were over 21. There were severe limitations surrounding the meaning of 'private'.

1986 Public Order Act

Created an offence for behaviour likely to cause a breach of the peace and disorderly conduct, and criminalised public affection for which heterosexual people would not be prosecuted.

1988 Local Government Act

(Section 28) A Local Authority shall not:

(a) intentionally promote homosexuality or publish material with the intention of promoting homosexuality;
(b) promote the teaching in any maintained school of the acceptability of homosexuality as a pretended family relationship

Nothing above shall be taken to prohibit the doing of anything for the purpose of treating or preventing the spread of disease.

1990 The Human Fertilisation and Embryology Act

Artificial insemination only provided if the need of that child for a father is considered; in practice it often excluded lesbians.

1994 Criminal Justice Act

The Act lowered the age of consent for gay men from 21 to 18, but did not remove other restrictions from the 1967 Act. A new offence of abuse of trust was introduced. Sexual relationships, whether heterosexual or homosexual, between young people aged 16–18 and adults in a position of authority, like teachers, were made unlawful. Same-sex sexual behaviour in the armed forces was no longer treated as a criminal offence. The first attempt to reduce the age of consent was in 1977.

1994 Homosexual Panic Defence

A homosexual panic defence, or Portsmouth defence, is a variation on the defence of provocation, a defence that only applies on a charge of murder.
    The defence was used in the case of Delamotta.

1997 Sexual Offenders Act

This Act required courts to place convicted sex offenders on a register. Men convicted of offences (including the younger person) before the lowering of the age of consent did not have their convictions quashed.

1999 Immigration policy

Changes mean that the probationary period that same-sex couples need to fulfil is reduced from four to two years.

2000 ACPO Guidelines for hate crimes.

The Association of Chief Police Officers (ACPO) produced a manual for the police service's approach to identifying and combating hate crime towards LGB people.

2000 Removal of the ban on LGB serving in the armed forces

This followed a judgement by the European Court of Human Rights which declared that discharging lesbians, gay men and bisexuals from the military forces because of their sexual identity violated Article 8 of the Convention – the right to a private life.

2000 Sexual Offences Bill

The age of consent for gay men was lowered to 16: this is now the same as for heterosexuals. Because of fierce opposition in the House of Lords, this legislation was passed by use of the Parliament Act in January 2001.

2001 Criminal Injuries Compensation

The scheme was revised by the Home Office to include long-term same-sex partners as qualifying relatives in fatal accidents.

2002 Adoption and Children Act

Although there has never been a law preventing LGB individuals from adopting children, there were a number of government circulars which suggested that LGB people were not suitable as parents. In practice, LGBs could adopt as single people, but could not apply to jointly adopt. The Act introduced provisions to enable same-sex couples to apply to jointly adopt children.

2002 Housing Law (*Ghaidan vs. Mendoza*)

This Law Lords judgement gave the right to same-sex couples to succeed to a tenancy in the event of the death of a partner. It stated: a person who had lived in a permanent homosexual relationship with the original tenant of rented accommodation could succeed, on the partner's death, to the tenancy and become a protected statutory tenant as the 'surviving spouse of the late partner'.

2003 Sexual Offences Act

The offences of gross indecency and buggery which particularly target gay men have been deleted from the statutes. There is a concern regarding a new offence of 'sexual activity in a public lavatory'. The Act criminalises sexual behaviour that a person knew, or ought to have known, was likely to cause distress, alarm or offence to others in a public place. Some gay men are worried that this offence will allow the police to continue to stigmatise them.

2003 Criminal Justice Act

This legislation does not create an offence for homophobic assault. However, it ensures that where an assault involved or was motivated by hostility or prejudice based on sexual orientation (actual or perceived) the judge is required to treat this as an aggravating factor. Section 146 of the Act was implemented in 2005 allowing courts to impose tougher sentences.

2003 Gender Recognition Act

This legislation allows transgender people to have their birth certificates altered to show their current gender status.

2003 Local Government Act

The provisions of the 1988 Local Government Act (including section 28) were repealed.

2003 Employment Equality (Sexual Orientation) Regulations

The new laws will prevent employers refusing to employ people because of their sexual identity and also protect workers from direct abuse and homophobia from colleagues. Employers will have to ensure that benefits given to opposite-sex partners can also be claimed by same-sex partners (unless the benefit is offered only to married couples).

2004 Domestic Violence, Crime and Victims Act

The Act recognises for the first time that same-sex couples experience domestic abuse. The Safety & Justice White Paper was the government's consultation document which proposed the main provisions on domestic violence under the three key headings of prevention, protection, justice and support.

2004 Fairness For All (White Paper)

The government sets out its intention to establish a new Commission for Equality and Human Rights covering all areas of inequality in terms of race, gender, disability, sexual identity, age and religion.

2004 Civil Partnership Act

The Act provides same-sex couples who form a civil partnership with parity of treatment in a wide range of legal matters with those opposite-sex couples who enter into a civil marriage. Provisions in the Act include:

- a duty to provide reasonable maintenance for the civil partner and any children of the family;
- civil partners to be assessed in the same way as spouses for child support;
- equitable treatment for the purposes of life assurance;
- employment and pension benefits;
- recognition under intestacy rules;
- access to fatal accidents compensation;
- protection from domestic violence;
- recognition for immigration and nationality purposes.

The legislation was implemented on 5 December 2005 and (with the 15-day waiting period) the first Civil Partnerships were registered on 21 December 2005.

2005 Equality Bill

An amendment has been made to the Equality Bill which will prohibit discrimination in the provision of goods and services to LGB people.

Appendix B

Abbreviations

ACPO	Association of Chief Police Officers
AIDS	Acquired Immune Deficiency Syndrome
Al-Fatiha	Gay, lesbian, bisexual and transgender Muslim association
APA	American Psychological Association
BMA	British Medical Association
BMJ	British Medical Journal
BSA	British Sociological Association
BSE	Breast self-examination
BV	Bacterial vaginosis (a sexually transmitted infection)
CEHR	Commission for Equality and Human Rights
CPS	Crown Prosecution Service
CRE	Commission for Racial Equality
CSP	Cervical Screening Programme
DFES	Department for Education and Science
DH	Department of Health
Diva	UK lesbian magazine
DRC	Disability Rights Commission
DSM	Diagnostic and Statistical Manual
DTI	Department of Trade and Industry
EER (SO)	Employment Equality Regulations (Sexual Orientation) 2003
EOC	Equal Opportunities Commission
EU	European Union
FGM	Female genital mutilation
FtM	Female to male (transsexual people)
Galop	LGBT anti-violence & police monitoring organisation
GID	Gender identity dysphoria
GLAM	Gay and Lesbian Arts and Media (now closed)
GP	General practitioner
GUM	Genito-urinary medicine
HBIGDA	Harry Benjamin International Gender Dysphoria Association
HIV	Human immunodeficiency virus (linked to AIDS)
HPV	Human papilloma virus (linked to cervical cancer)
Indico Trust	LGBT charitable organisation established to commission research
KISS	London-based South Asian lesbian group
LFS	Labour Force Survey
LGB(T)	Lesbians, Gay men, Bisexual and (Transgender)
LHCS	Lesbians and Health Care Survey
Mencap	UK learning disability charity
MIND	UK mental health charity
MP	Member of Parliament

MSM	Men who have sex with men
MtF	Male to female (transsexual people)
NACRO	National Association for the Care and Resettlement of Offenders
NATSAL	National Survey of Sexual Attitudes and Lifestyles – a UK population-based study conducted in 1990 and 2000
NHSLS	National Health and Social Life Survey – a US population-based study
Naz Project	Charity providing sexual health education, HIV/AIDS programmes for South Asian, Middle Eastern, North African LGB people
NGMSS	National Gay Men's Sex Survey
NHS	National Health Service
OPCS	Office of Population Censuses and Surveys
PFC	Press for Change – campaigning group for trans people
RCN	Royal College of Nursing
RDD	Random digit-dialling
Regard	National organisation of disabled lesbians, gay men bisexuals and transgender people
Safra Project	Resource project for lesbian, bisexual and transgender Muslim women
SRE	Sex and relationships education guidance
SRS	Sex reassignment surgery
STI	Sexually transmitted infection
UAI	Unprotected anal intercourse
WEU	Women and Equality Unit

References

ACPO (2000) *Breaking the Power of Fear and Hate: Identifying and Combating Hate Crime*, London: Association of Chief Police Officers.

Adams, C. L. J. and Kimmel, D. C. (1997) 'Exploring the Lives of Older African American Gay Men' (pp. 132–51), in B. Greene (ed.), *Ethnic and Cultural Diversity among Lesbians and Gay Men*, Thousand Oaks, CA: Sage Publications.

Arabsheibani, G. R., Marin, A. and Wadsworth, J. (2004) 'In the Pink: Homosexual–Heterosexual Wage Differentials in the UK', *International Journal of Manpower*, 25, 3/4: 343–54.

Audit Commission (2002) *Directions in Diversity: Current Opinion and Good Practice*, London: Audit Commission.

Bacchi, C. L. (1990) *Same Difference: Feminism and Sexual Difference*, Sydney: Allen & Unwin.

Badgett, L. and Hyman, P. (1998) 'Towards Lesbian, Gay and Bisexual Perspectives in Economics: Why and How They May Make a Difference', *Feminist Economics*, 4, 2: 49–54.

Badgett, M. V. L. (1998) *Income Inflation: the Myth of Affluence Among Gay, Lesbian and Bisexual Americans*, retrieved 19 July 2005 from http://www.thetaskforce.org.

Bailey, J. V., Farquhar, C. and Owen, C. (2004), 'Bacterial Vaginosis in Lesbians and Bisexual Women', *Sexually Transmitted Diseases*, 31, 11: 691–4.

Bailey, J. V., Kavanagh, J., Owen, C., McClean, K. A. and Skinner, C. J. (2000) 'Lesbians and Cervical Screening', *British Journal of General Practice*, 50: 481–2.

Battle, J., Cohen, C., Warren, D., Fergerson, G. and Audam, S. (2002) 'Say It Loud: I'm Black and I'm Proud; Black Pride Survey 2000', New York: The Policy Institute of the National Gay and Lesbian Task Force.

Baum, M., Saunders, C. and Meredith, S. (1994) *Breast Cancer: a Guide for Every Woman*, Oxford: Oxford University Press.

Bayliss, K. (2000) 'Social Work Values, Anti-discriminatory Practice and Working with Older Lesbian Service Users', *Social Work Education*, 19, 1: 45–53.

Beckett, C. and Macey, M. (2001) 'Race, Gender and Sexuality: the Oppression of Multiculturalism', *Women's Studies International Forum*, 24, 3–4: 309–19.

Beehler, G. P. (2001) 'Confronting the Culture of Medicine: Gay Men's Experiences with Primary Care Physicians', *Journal of the Gay & Lesbian Medical Association*, 5, 4: 135–44.

Ben-Ari, A. T. (2001) 'Homosexuality and Heterosexism: Views from Academics in the Helping Professions', *British Journal of Social Work*, 31: 119–31.

Bene, E. (1965a), 'On the Genesis of Female Homosexuality', *British Journal of Psychiatry*, 111: 815–21.

Bene, E. (1965b) 'On the Genesis of Male Homosexuality: an Attempt at Clarifying the Role of the Parents', *British Journal of Psychiatry*, 111: 803–13.

Bergmark, K. H. (1999) 'Drinking in the Swedish Gay and Lesbian Community', *Drug and Alcohol Dependence*, 56, 2: 133–43.

Bhugra, D. (1997) 'Coming Out by South Asian Gay Men in the United Kingdom', *Archives of Sexual Behavior*, 26, 5: 547–57.

Birke, L. (2002) 'Unusual Fingers: Scientific Studies of Sexuality' (pp. 55–71), in D. Richardson and S. Seidman (eds), *Handbook of Lesbian & Gay Studies*, London: Sage Publications.

Black, D., Gates, G., Sanders, S. and Taylor, L. (2000) 'Demographics of the Gay and Lesbian Population in the United States: Evidence from Available Systematic Data Sources', *Demography*, 37, 2: 139–54.

Blumenfeld, W. J. (ed.) (1992) *Homophobia: How We All Pay the Price*, Boston, MA: Beacon Press.

BMA (2005) *Sexual Orientation in the Workplace*, London: BMA.

Boehmer, U. (2002) 'Twenty Years of Public Health Research: Inclusion of Lesbian, Gay, Bisexual, and Transgender Populations', *American Journal of Public Health*, 92, 7: 1125–30.

Boehmer, U. and Case, P. (2004) 'Physicians Don't Ask, Sometimes Patients Tell: Disclosure of Sexual Orientation among Women with Breast Cancer', *Cancer*, 101, 8: 1882–9.

Bowleg, L., Craig, M. L. and Burkholder, G. (2004) 'Rising and Surviving: a Conceptual Model of Active Coping among Black Lesbians', *Cultural Diversity and Ethnic Minority Psychology*, 10, 3: 229–40.

Box, V. (1998) 'Cervical Screening: the Knowledge and Opinions of Black and Ethnic Minority Women and of Health Advocates in East London', *Health Education Journal*, 57: 3–15.

Bradford, J., Honnold, J. A. and Ryan, C. (1997) 'Disclosure of Sexual Orientation in Survey Research on Women', *Journal of the Gay & Lesbian Medical Association*, 1, 3: 169–77.

Brickell, C. (2001) 'Whose "Special Treatment"? Heterosexism and the Problems with Liberalism', *Sexualities*, 4, 2: 211–35.

Bridges, S. K., Selvidge, M. M. D. and Matthews, C. R. (2003) 'Lesbian Women of Color: Therapeutic Issues and Challenges', *Journal of Multicultural Counseling & Development*, 31, 2: 113–30.

Brogan, D., Frank, E., Elon, L. and O' Hanlan, K. A. (2001) 'Methodologic Concerns in Defining Lesbian for Health Research', *Epidemiology*, 12, 1: 109–13.

Brown, H. C. (1998) *Social Work and Sexuality: Working with Lesbians and Gay Men*, Basingstoke: Macmillan.

Brownworth, V. (1993) 'The Other Epidemic: Lesbians and Breast Cancer', *OUT*: 61–3.

Bullough, V. L. (2000) 'Transgenderism and the Concept of Gender', *The International Journal of Transgenderism: Special Issue: What is Transgender?* 4, 3. Available at http://www.symposion.com/ijt/gilbert/bullough.htm.

Burke, L. K. and Follingstad, D. R. (1999) 'Violence in Lesbian and Gay Relationships: Theory, Prevalence and Correlational Factors', *Clinical Psychology Review*, 19, 5: 487–512.

Cant, B. (1999) 'Primary Care Needs of Gay and Bisexual Men and Their Perceptions of Primary Care Practice', unpublished report, available from Bromley Health Authority, Global House, 10 Station Approach, Hayes, Kent, BR2 7EH.

Cant, B. (2003) *Are They There? Report of Research into Health Issues Relating to Lesbian, Gay and Bisexual Young People in Lambeth, Southwark and Lewisham*, South Bank University, London: Faculty of Health.

Carroll, R. (1999) 'Soho Bombing: a Balmy Evening that Ended in Death', *The Guardian*, 1 May: 3.

Cass, V. C. (1979) 'Homosexual Identity Formation: a Theoretical Model', *Journal of Homosexuality*, 4, 3: 219–35.

Champion, J. D., Wilford, K., Shain, R. N. and Piper, J. M. (2005) 'Risk and Protective Behaviours of Bisexual Minority Women: a Qualitative Analysis', *International Nursing Review*, 52, 2: 115–22.

Chan, C. S. (1996) 'Combating Heterosexism in Educational Institutions: Structural Changes and Strategies' (pp. 20–35), in E. Rothblum and L. A. Bond (eds), *Preventing Heterosexism and Homophobia*, Thousand Oaks, CA: Sage.

Chiu, L.-F. and Knight, D. (1999) 'How Useful are Focus Groups for Obtaining the Views of Minority Groups?' (pp. 99–112), in R. Barbour and J. Kitzinger (eds), *Developing Focus Group Research: Politics, Theory & Practice*, London: Sage Publications.

Chu, S., Buehler, J., Fleming, P. and Berkelman, R. (1990) 'Epidemiology of Reported Cases of AIDS in Lesbians', *American Journal of Public Health*, 80: 1380–1.

Chung, Y. B. and Katayama, M. (1998) 'Ethnic and Sexual Identity Development of Asian-American Lesbian and Gay Adolescents', *Professional School Counseling*, 1, 3: 21.

Clarke, V. (1999) ' "God made Adam and Eve, not Adam and Steve": Lesbian and Gay Parenting on Talk Shows', *Lesbian & Gay Psychology Review*, 1, 1: 7–17.

Clarke, V. (2001) 'Lesbian and Gay Parenting: Resistance and Normalisation', *Lesbian & Gay Psychology Review*, 2, 1: 3–8.

Clutterbuck, D. J., Gorman, D., McMillan, A., Lewis, R. and Macintyre, C. C. (2001) 'Substance Use and Unsafe Sex amongst Homosexual Men in Edinburgh', *AIDS Care*, 13, 4: 527–35.

Cochran, S. D., Mays, V. M., Bowen, D., Gage, S., Bybee, D., Roberts, S. J., Goldstein, R. S., Robison, A., Rankow, E. J. and White, J. (2001) 'Cancer-related Risk Indicators and Preventive Screening Behaviors among Lesbians and Bisexual Women', *American Journal of Public Health*, 91, 4: 591–7.

Cochran, S. D., Mays, V. M. and Sullivan, J. G. (2003) 'Prevalence of Mental Disorders, Psychological Distress, and Mental Health Services Use among Lesbian, Gay, and Bisexual Adults in the United States', *Journal of Consulting & Clinical Psychology*, 71, 1: 53–61.

Coia, N., John, S., Dobbie, F., Bruce, S., McGranachan, M. and Simons, L. (2002) 'Something to Tell You': a Health Needs Assessment of Young Gay, Lesbian and Bisexual People in Glasgow*, Glasgow: Greater Glasgow Health Board.

Cole Wilson, O. and Allen, C. (1994) 'The Black Perspective' (pp. 112–36), in E. Healey and A. Mason (eds), *Stonewall 25: the Making of the Lesbian and Gay Community in Britain*, London: Virago Press.

Collins, M. (2002) 'Sampling for UK Telephone Surveys' (pp. 85–9), in D. de Vaus (ed.), *Social Surveys: Sage Benchmarks in Social Research Methods*, London: Sage Publications.

Coney, S. (1995) *The Menopause Industry*, London: Women's Press.

Consolacion, T. B., Russell, S. T. and Sue, S. (2004) 'Sex, Race/Ethnicity, and Romantic Attractions: Multiple Minority Status Adolescents and Mental Health', *Cultural Diversity and Ethnic Minority Psychology*, 10, 3: 200–14.

Cooper, D., Carabine, J. and Munro, S. (2004) *The Changing Politics of Lesbian and Gay Equality in Local Government 1990–2001*, Swindon: Economic and Social Research Council.

Crawford, T., Geraghty, W., Street, K. and Simonoff, E. (2003) 'Staff Knowledge and Attitudes Towards Deliberate Self-Harm in Adolescents', *Journal of Adolescence*, 26, 5: 623–33.

Creith, E. (1996) *Undressing Lesbian Sex: Popular Images, Private Acts and Public Consequences*, London: Cassell.

Dalrymple, J. and Burke, B. (2001) *Anti-Oppressive Practice: Social Care and the Law*, Buckingham: Open University Press.

Dang, A. and Frazer, S. (2005), 'Found: 85,000 Black Gay Households', *Gay & Lesbian Review Worldwide*, 12, 1: 29–30.

Davies, P. (1992) 'The Role of Disclosure in Coming Out among Gay Men' (pp. 75–83), in K. Plummer (ed.), *Modern Homosexualities: Fragments of Lesbian and Gay Experience*, London: Routledge.

De Cecco, J. P. (1981) 'Definition and Meaning of Sexual Orientation', *Journal of Homosexuality*, 6, 4: 51–65.

de Gruchy, J. and Fish, J. (2004) 'Doctors' Involvement in Human Rights Abuses of Men Who Have Sex with Men in Egypt', *The Lancet*, 363: 1903.

Dean, L., Meyer, I. H., Robinson, K., Sell, R. L., Sember, R., Silenzio, V. M. B., Bowen, D. J., Bradford, J., Rothblum, E., White, J., Dunn, P., Lawrence, A., Wolfe, D. and Xavier, J. (2000) 'Lesbian, Gay, Bisexual, and Transgender Health: Findings and Concerns', *Journal of the Gay & Lesbian Medical Association*, 4, 3: 102–51.

Di Ceglie, D., Freedman, D., McPherson, S. and Richardson, P. (2002) 'Children and Adolescents Referred to a Specialist Gender Identity Development Service: Clinical Features and Demographic Characteristics', *The International Journal of Transgenderism*, 6, 1. Available at http://www.symposion.com/ijt/ijtvo06no01_01.htm.

Diamant, A. L., Wold, C., Spritzer, K. and Gelberg, L. (2000) 'Health Behaviors, Health Status, and Access to and Use of Health Care: a Population-based Study of Lesbian, Bisexual and Heterosexual Women', *Archives of Family Medicine*, 9, 10: 1043–51.

Diamant, A. L. and Wold, C. (2003) 'Sexual Orientation and Variation in Physical and Mental Health Status among Women', *Journal of Women's Health*, 12, 1: 41–9.

Diaz, R. M., Ayala, G., Bein, D. E., Henne, J. and Marin, B. V. (2001) 'The Impact of Homophobia, Poverty, and Racism on the Mental Health of Gay and Bisexual Latino Men: Findings from 3 US Cities', *American Journal of Public Health*, 91, 6: 927–32.

Diaz, R. M., Ayala, G. and Bein, E. (2004) 'Sexual Risk as an Outcome of Social Oppression: Data from a Probability Sample of Latino Gay Men in Three US Cities', *Cultural Diversity and Ethnic Minority Psychology*, 10, 3: 255–67.

Dibble, S. L. and Roberts, S. A. (2002) 'A Comparison of Breast Cancer Diagnosis and Treatment between Lesbian and Heterosexual Women', *Journal of the Gay & Lesbian Medical Association*, 6, 1: 9–17.

Dodds, J. P., Nardone, A., Mercey, D. E. and Johnson, A. M. (2005) 'Increase in High Risk Sexual Behaviour among Homosexual Men, London 1996–8: Cross-sectional, Questionnaire Study', *British Medical Journal*, 320: 1510–11.

Dominelli, L. (2002) *Anti-Oppressive Social Work Theory and Practice*, Basingstoke: Palgrave Macmillan.

Duncker, P. (1993) 'Heterosexuality: Fictional Agendas' (pp. 137–49), in S. Wilkinson and C. Kitzinger (eds), *Heterosexuality: a Feminism & Psychology Reader*, London: Sage.

Edelman, L. (1993) 'Tearooms and Sympathy, or, the Epistemology of the Water Closet' (pp. 553–74), in H. Abelove, M. A. Barale and D. M. Halperin (eds), *The Lesbian and Gay Studies Reader*, New York: Routledge.

Ekins, R. and King, D. (1997) 'Blending Genders: Contributions to the Emerging Field of Transgender Studies', *The International Journal of Transgenderism*, 1, 1.

Elford, J., Bolding, G., Maguire, M. and Sherr, L. (2000) 'Do Gay Men Discuss HIV Risk Reduction with their GP?' *AIDS Care*, 12, 3: 287–90.

Eliason, M. J. (2000) 'Substance Abuse Counselors' Attitudes Regarding Lesbian, Gay, Bisexual, and Transgendered Clients', *Journal of Substance Abuse*, 12, 4: 311–28.

Eliason, M. and Schope, R. (2001) 'Does "Don't Ask Don't Tell" Apply to Health Care? Lesbian, Gay and Bisexual People's Disclosure to Health Care Providers', *Journal of the Gay & Lesbian Medical Association*, 5, 4: 125–34.

Ellingson, L. A. and Yarber, W. L. (1997) 'Breast Self-Examination, the Health Belief Model, and Sexual Orientation in Women', *Journal of Sex Education & Therapy*, 22, 3: 19–24.

Ellis, B. (1995) *The Experiences of Disabled Women*, York: Joseph Rowntree Foundation.

Ellis, V. and High, S. (2004) 'Something More to Tell You: Gay, Lesbian or Bisexual Young People's Experiences of Secondary Schooling', *British Educational Research Journal*, 30, 2: 213–25.

Emmanuel, J., Potts, L., Thomson, L. and Twomey, M. (1989) 'Choice and Control in Breast Disease' (pp. 535–56), in A. Phillips and J. Rakusen (eds), *Our Bodies, Our Selves: a Health Book by and for Women*, London: Penguin Books.

Esterberg, K. G. (2002) 'The Bisexual Menace: Or, Will the Real Bisexual Please Stand Up?' (pp. 215–27), in D. Richardson and S. Seidman (eds), *Handbook of Lesbian & Gay Studies*, London: Sage Publications.

Ettorre, E. (ed.) (2005) *Making Lesbians Visible in the Substance Abuse Field*, Binghampton, NY: Haworth Press.

Eyler, E. A. and Whittle, S. (2001) 'FTM Breast Cancer: Community Awareness and Illustrative Cases', paper presented at the XVII Harry Benjamin International Gender Dysphoria Association Symposium, 31 October–4 November 2001, Galveston, Texas, USA.

Faderman, L. (1992) *Odd Girls and Twilight Lovers: a History of Lesbian Life in Twentieth-Century America*, Harmondsworth: Penguin.

Fee, E., Brown, T. and Laylor, J. (2003) 'One Size Does Not Fit All in the Transgender Community', *American Journal of Public Health*, 93, 6: 899–900.

Feinberg, L. (2001) 'Trans Health Crisis: For Us It's Life or Death', *American Journal of Public Health*, 91, 6: 897.

Feldman, J. and Bockting, W. (2001) 'Primary Care of the Transgender Patient', paper presented at the XVII Harry Benjamin International Gender Dysphoria Association Symposium, 31 October–4 November, Galveston, Texas, USA.

Fine, M. and Addelston, J. (1996) 'Containing Questions of Gender and Power: the Discursive Limits of "Sameness" and "Difference" ' (pp. 66–86), in S. Wilkinson (ed.), *Feminist Social Psychologies: International Perspectives*, Buckingham: Open University Press.

Finlon, C. (2002) 'Health Care for All Lesbian, Gay, Bisexual, and Transgender Populations', *Journal of Gay and Lesbian Social Services*, 14, 3: 109–16.

Fish, J. (1993) 'Researching Lesbians' Identities', unpublished MA dissertation, University of Wolverhampton.

Fish, J. (1999) 'Sampling Lesbians: How to Get 1000 Lesbians to Complete a Questionnaire', *Feminism & Psychology*, 9, 2: 229–38.

Fish, J. (2000) 'Sampling Issues in Lesbian and Gay Psychology: Challenges in Achieving Diversity', *Lesbian & Gay Psychology Review*, 1, 2: 32–8.

Fish, J. (2002) 'Lesbians and Health Care: a National Survey of Lesbians' Health Behaviour and Experiences', unpublished PhD: Loughborough University.

Fish, J. (2005) *The Health and Health Care Needs of LGBT People*, retrieved 21 October 2005 from http://www.pohg.org.uk.

Fish, J. and Anthony, D. (2005) 'UK National Lesbians and Health Care Survey', *Women and Health*, 41, 3: 27–45.

Fish, J. and Wilkinson, S. (2003a) 'Understanding Lesbians' Healthcare Behaviour: the Case of Breast Self-Examination', *Social Science & Medicine*, 56, 2: 235–45.

Fish, J. and Wilkinson, S. (2003b) 'Explaining Lesbians' Practice of Breast Self-Examination: Results from a UK Survey of Lesbian Health', *Health Education Journal*, 62, 4: 304–15.

Flowers, P. and Buston, K. (2001) ' "I Was Terrified of Being Different": Exploring Gay Men's Accounts of Growing-up in a Heterosexist Society', *Journal of Adolescence*, 24, 1: 51–65.

Flowers, P., Duncan, B. and Knussen, C. (2003) 'Re-appraising HIV Testing: an Exploration of the Psychological Costs and Benefits Associated with Learning One's HIV Status in a Purposive Sample of Scottish Gay Men', *British Journal of Health Psychology*, 8 (Part 2): 179–94.

French, S. A., Story, M., Remafedi, G., Resnick, M. D. and Blum, R. W. (1996) 'Sexual Orientation and Prevalence of Body Dissatisfaction and Eating Disordered Behaviors: a Population-Based Study of Adolescents', *International Journal of Eating Disorders*, 19, 2: 119–26.

Frye, M. (1998) 'Oppression' (pp. 146–9), in P. S. Rothenberg (ed.), *Race, Class, and Gender in the United States: an Integrated Study*, New York: St. Martin's Press.

Gadd, D., Farrall, S., Dallimore, D. and Lombard, N. (2002) *Domestic Abuse Against Men in Scotland*, Edinburgh: Scottish Executive.

Galop (1998) *Telling It Like It Is . . . Lesbian, Gay and Bisexual Youth Speak Out on Homophobic Violence*, London: Galop.

Galop (2001) *The Low Down, Black Lesbians, Gay Men and Bisexual People Talk about Their Experiences and Needs*, London: Galop.

Gerstel, C. J., Feraios, A. J. and Herdt, G. (1989) 'Widening Circles: an Ethnographic Profile of a Youth Group' (pp. 75–92), in G. Herdt (ed.), *Gay and Lesbian Youth*, New York: Haworth Press.

Gillespie-Sells, K., Hill, M. and Robbins, B. (eds) (1998) *She Dances to Different Drums: Research into Disabled Women's Sexuality*, London: The King's Fund.

Golden, C. R. (2000) 'Still Seeing Differently, After All These Years', *Feminism & Psychology*, 10, 1: 30–5.

Gomez, J. L. and Smith, B. (1994) 'Taking the Home out of Homophobia: Black Lesbian Health' (pp. 185–204), in M. Wilson (ed.), *Healthy and Wise: the Essential Health Handbook for Black Women*, London: Virago Press.

Greene, B. (2000) 'African-American Lesbian and Bisexual Women', *Journal of Social Issues*, 56, 2: 239–49.

Greene, B. (2003) 'Beyond Heterosexism and Across the Cultural Divides – Developing an Inclusive Lesbian, Gay and Bisexual Psychology: a Look to the Future' (pp. 67–93), in L. Garnets and D. C. Kimmel (eds), *Psychological Perspectives on Lesbian, Gay, and Bisexual Experiences*, New York, NY: Columbia University Press.

Gross, L. (1993) *Contested Closets: the Politics and Ethics of Outing*, Minnesota: University of Minnesota Press.

Gruskin, E. P. (1999) *Treating Lesbians and Bisexual Women: Challenges and Strategies for Health Professionals*, Thousand Oaks, CA: Sage Publications.

Gruskin, E. P., Hart, S., Gordon, N. and Ackerson, L. (2001) 'Patterns of Cigarette Smoking and Alcohol Use among Lesbians and Bisexual Women Enrolled in a Large Health Maintenance Organization', *American Journal of Public Health*, 91, 6: 976–9.

Harry, J. (1993) 'Being Out: a General Model', *Journal of Homosexuality*, 26, 10: 25–39.

Hart, G. J., Williamson, L. M., Flowers, P., Frankis, J. S. and Der, G. J. (2002) 'Gay Men's HIV Testing Behaviour in Scotland', *AIDS Care*, 14, 5: 665–74.

Haynes, S. (1992) 'Are Lesbians at High Risk of Breast Cancer?' Paper presented at the 14th National Gay and Lesbian Health Foundation Conference, Los Angeles, CA.

Heaphy, B., Yip, A. and Thompson, D. (2003) *Lesbian, Gay and Bisexual Lives over 50: a Report on the Project 'The Social and Policy Implications of Non-Heterosexual Ageing'*, Nottingham Trent University: York House Publications.

Heckathorn, D. D. (2002) 'Respondent-Driven Sampling II: Deriving Valid Population Estimates from Chain-Referral Samples of Hidden Populations', *Social Problems*, 49, 1: 11–34.

Henderson, L., Reid, D., Hickson, F., McLean, S., Cross, J. and Weatherburn, P. (2002) *First, Service: Relationships, Sex and Health among Lesbian and Bisexual Women*, Sigma Research.

Hensher, P. (2005) 'Gay for Today', *The Guardian*, 24 November: 22–3.

Herek, G. M. (2004) 'Beyond "Homophobia": Thinking about Sexual Prejudice and Stigma in the Twenty-First Century', *Sexuality Research & Social Policy*, 1, 2: 6–24.

Herrell, R., Goldberg, J., True, W. R., Ramakrishnan, V., Lyons, M., Eisen, S. and Tsuang, M. T. (1999) 'Sexual Orientation and Suicidality: a Co-Twin Control Study in Adult Men', *Archives of General Psychiatry*, 56: 867–74.

Hicks, S. (2000) ' "Good Lesbian, Bad Lesbian. . .": Regulating Heterosexuality in Fostering and Adoption Assessments', *Child & Family Social Work*, 5, 2: 157–68.

Hickson, F., Reid, D., Weatherburn, P., Henderson, L. and Stephens, M. (1998) *Making Data Count: Findings from the National Gay Men's Sex Survey 1997*, London: CHAPS Partnership, The Terence Higgins Trust. Available from: Sigma Research, 64 Eurolink Centre, 49 Effra Road, London. SW2 1BZ.

Hickson, F., Weatherburn, P., Reid, D. and Stephens, M. (2002) *Out and About: Findings from the United Kingdom Gay Men's Sex Survey 2002*, Sigma Research.

Hickson, F., Reid, D., Weatherburn, P., Stephens, M., Nutland, W. and Boakye, P. (2004) 'HIV, Sexual Risk and Ethnicity Among Men in England Who Have Sex with Men', *Sexually Transmitted Infections*, 80: 443–50.

Hinchliff, S., Gott, M. and Galena, E. (2005) ' "I Daresay I Might Find It Embarrassing": General Practitioners' Perspectives on Discussing Sexual Health

Issues with Lesbian and Gay Patients', *Health & Social Care in the Community*, 13, 4: 345–53.

Hitchcock, J. M. and Wilson, H. S. (1992) 'Personal Risk Taking: Lesbian Self-Disclosure of Sexual Orientation to Professional Health Care Providers', *Nursing Research*, 41, 3: 178–83.

Hopkins, J. H. (1969) 'The Lesbian Personality', *British Journal of Psychiatry*, 115: 1433–6.

Hughes, D. (2004) 'Disclosure of Sexual Preferences and Lesbian, Gay, and Bisexual Practitioners', *British Medical Journal*, 328, 7450: 1211–12.

Hughes, T. L. (2003) 'Lesbians' Drinking Patterns: Beyond the Data', *Substance Use & Misuse*, 38, 11–13: 1739–58.

Hughes, T. L., Johnson, T. and Wilsnack, S. C. (2001) 'Sexual Assault and Alcohol Abuse: a Comparison of Lesbians and Heterosexual Women', *Journal of Substance Abuse*, 13, 4: 515–32.

Johnson, A. M., Mercer, C. H., Erens, B., Copas, A. J., McManus, S., Wellings, K., Fenton, K. A., Korovessis, C., Macdowall, W., Nanchahal, K., Purdon, S. and Field, J. (2001) 'Sexual Behaviour in Britain: Partnerships, Practices and HIV Risk Behaviours', *The Lancet*, 358: 1835–42.

Johnson, C. (2002) 'Heteronormative Citizenship and the Politics of Passing', *Sexualities*, 5, 3: 317–36.

Kaminski, P. L., Chapman, B. J., Haynes, S. D. and Own, L. (2005) 'Body Image, Eating Behaviors, and Attitudes toward Exercise among Gay and Straight Men', *Eating Behaviors*, 6, 3: 179–87.

Kenyon, F. E. (1968) 'Studies in Female Homosexuality: IV Social and Psychiatric Aspects', *British Journal of Psychiatry*, 114: 1337–50.

Kitchen, G. (2003) *Social Care Needs of Older Gay Men and Lesbians on Merseyside*, Liverpool: Sefton Pensioners Advocacy Centre.

Keogh, P., Henderson, L. and Dodds, C. (2004a) *Ethnic Minority Gay Men Redefining Community, Restoring Identity*, Sigma Research.

Keogh, P., Weatherburn, P., Henderson, L., Reid, D., Dodds, C. and Hickson, F. (2004b) *Doctoring Gay Men: Exploring the Contribution of General Practice*, Sigma Research.

Kessler, S. and McKenna, W. (2000) 'Gender Construction in Everyday Life', *Feminism & Psychology*, 10, 1: 11–29.

King, M., McKeown, E., Warner, J., Ramsay, A., Johnson, K., Cort, C., Wright, L. et al. (2003) 'Mental Health and Quality of Life of Gay Men and Lesbians in England and Wales: Controlled, Cross-sectional Study', *British Journal of Psychiatry*, 183, 6: 552–8.

Kinsey, A. C., Pomeroy, W. B. and Martin, C. E. (1948) *Sexual Behavior in the Human Male*, Philadelphia: W.B. Saunders Company.

Kinsey, A. C., Pomeroy, W. B., Martin, C. E. and Gebhard, P. H. (1953) *Sexual Behavior in the Human Female*, Philadelphia: W.B. Saunders Company.

Kitzinger, C. (1996) 'Speaking of Oppression: Psychology, Politics, and the Power of Language' (pp. 3–19), in E. Rothblum and L. A. Bond (eds), *Preventing Heterosexism and Homophobia*, Thousand Oaks, CA: Sage.

Kitzinger, C. and Perkins, R. (1993) *Changing Our Minds: Lesbian Feminism and Psychology*, London: Onlywomen Press.

Kitzinger, C. and Wilkinson, S. (1993) 'Theorizing Heterosexuality' (pp. 1–32), in S. Wilkinson and C. Kitzinger (eds), *Heterosexuality: a Feminism & Psychology Reader*, London: Sage.

Koh, A. S. and Diamant, A. L. (2000) 'Use of Preventive Health Behaviors by Lesbian, Bisexual and Heterosexual Women: Questionnaire Survey', *Western Journal of Medicine*, 172, 6: 379–84.

Kosofsky-Sedgwick, E. (1993) 'Epistemology of the Closet' (pp. 45–61), in H. Abelove, M. A. Barale and D. M. Halperin (eds), *The Lesbian and Gay Studies Reader*, London: Routledge.

Laird, N. (2004) *Exploring Biphobia: a Report on Participatory Workshops in Glasgow and Edinburgh*, retrieved 20 May 2005 from http://www.stonewall.org.uk/beyond_barriers.

Laird, N. and Aston, L. (2003) *Participatory Appraisal Transgender Research*, retrieved 21 March 2005 from http://www.beyondbarriers.org.uk.

Langley, J. (2001) 'Developing Anti-Oppressive Empowering Social Work Practice with Older Lesbian Women and Gay Men', *British Journal of Social Work*, 31, 6: 917–32.

Laumann, E. O., Gagnon, J. H., Michael, R. T. and Michaels, S. (1994) *The Social Organization of Sexuality: Sexual Practices in the United States*, Chicago: University of Chicago Press.

Lee, R. and Renzetti, C. (1993) 'The Problems of Researching Sensitive Topics' (pp. 3–13), in R. Lee and C. Renzetti (eds), *Researching Sensitive Topics*, Newbury Park, CA: Sage Publications.

Lemp, G. F., Jones, M., Kellog, T. A., Nieri, G., Anderson, L., Withum, D. and Katz, M. (1995) 'HIV Seroprevalence and Risk Behaviors among Lesbians and Bisexual Women in San Francisco and Berkeley, California', *American Journal of Public Health*, 85, 11: 1549–52.

LeVay, S. (1993) *The Sexual Brain*, Cambridge, MA: MIT Press.

Logan, J., Kershaw, S., Mills, S., Trotter, J. and Sinclair, M. (1996) *Confronting Prejudice: Lesbian and Gay Issues in Social Work Education*, Aldershot: Arena.

Lombardi, E. (2001) 'Enhancing Transgender Care', *American Journal of Public Health*, 96, 6: 869–72.

Love, S. (1995) *Dr Susan Love's Breast Book*, Reading, MA: Addison-Wesley Publishing Company.

Lupton, D. (1993) 'Risk as Moral Danger: the Social and Political Functions of Risk Discourse in Public Health', *International Journal of Health Services*, 23, 3: 425–35.

Lupton, D., McCarthy, S. and Chapman, S. (1995) ' "Panic Bodies": Discourses on Risk and HIV Antibody Testing', *Sociology of Health & Illness*, 17, 1: 89–108.

MacCallum, F. and Golombok, S. (2004) 'Children Raised in Fatherless Families from Infancy: a Follow-up of Children of Lesbian and Single Heterosexual Mothers at Early Adolescence', *Journal of Child Psychology & Psychiatry & Allied Disciplines*, 45, 8: 1407–19.

Malebranche, D. J., Peterson, J. L., Fullilove, R. E. and Stackhouse, R. W. (2004) 'Race and Sexual Identity: Perceptions About Medical Culture and Healthcare among Black Men Who Have Sex with Men', *Journal of the National Medical Association*, 96, 1: 97–107.

Markowe, L. A. (1996) *Redefining the Self: Coming out as Lesbian*, Cambridge: Polity Press.

Martin, J. L. and Dean, L. (1993) 'Developing a Community Sample of Gay Men for an Epidemiological Study of AIDS' (pp. 82–99), in C. Renzetti and R. Lee (eds), *Researching Sensitive Topics*, Newbury Park, CA: Sage Publications.

Martinson, J. C., Fisher, D. G. and DeLapp, T. D. (1996) 'Client Disclosure of Lesbianism: a Challenge for Health Care Providers', *Journal of Gay and Lesbian Social Services*, 4, 3: 81–94.

Mason, A. and Palmer, A. (1996) *Queer Bashing: a National Survey of Hate Crimes against Lesbians and Gay Men*, London: Stonewall.

Mason-John, V. (ed.) (1995) *Talking Black: Lesbians of African and Asian Descent Speak Out*, London: Cassell.

Matheson, J. and Summerfield, C. (2000) *Social Trends, 30*, Office for National Statistics. London: HMSO.

Matthews, A. K. and Hughes, T. L. (2001) 'Mental Health Service Use by African-American Women: Exploration of Subpopulation Differences', *Cultural Diversity and Ethnic Minority Psychology*, 7, 1: 75–87.

McCabe, S. E., Hughes, T. L. and Boyd, C. J. (2004) 'Substance Use and Misuse: Are Bisexual Women at Greater Risk?' *Journal of Psychoactive Drugs*, 36, 2: 217–25.

McClennen, J. C., Summers, A. B. and Daley, J. G. (2002) 'The Lesbian Partner Abuse Scale', *Research on Social Work Practice*, 12, 2: 277–92.

McDermott, L. (2004) 'Telling Lesbian Stories: Interviewing and the Class Dynamics of "Talk" ', *Women's Studies International Forum*, 27: 177–87.

McFarlane, L. (1998) *Diagnosis Homophobic: the Experiences of Lesbians, Gay Men and Bisexuals in Mental Health Services*, London: Pace.

McIntosh, P. (1998) 'White Privilege: Unpacking the Invisible Knapsack' (pp. 165–9), in P. S. Rothenberg (ed.), *Race, Class, and Gender in the United States: an Integrated Study*, New York, St. Martin's Press.

McKenna, W. and Kessler, S. (2000) 'Who Put the "Trans" in Transgender? Gender Theory and Everyday Life', *The International Journal of Transgenderism*, 4, 3. Available at http://www.symposion.com/ijt/gilbert/kessler.htm.

McKie, L. (1995) 'The Art of Surveillance or Reasonable Prevention? The Case for Cervical Screening', *Sociology of Health and Illness*, 17, 4: 441–57.

McKie, L. (1996), 'Women Hearing Men: the Cervical Smear Test and the Social Construction of Sexuality' (pp. 120–35), in J. Holland and L. Adkins (eds), *Sex, Sensibility and the Gendered Body*, Basingstoke: Macmillan.

Mclean, C., Campbell, C. and Cornish, F. (2003) 'African-Caribbean Interactions with Mental Health Services in the UK: Experiences and Expectations of Exclusion as (Re) Productive of Health Inequalities', *Social Science & Medicine*, 56, 3: 657–70.

McLean, C. and O'Connor, W. (2003) *Sexual Orientation Research Phase 2: the Future of LGBT Research – Perspectives of Community Organisations*, Edinburgh: Scottish Executive.

McLean, G. (2004) 'Words That Inspire the Killer Deeds: Homophobic Politicians, Singers and Journalists Share the Blame', *The Guardian*, 3 November: 26.

Meyer, I. H. (2001) 'Why Lesbian, Gay, Bisexual, and Transgender Public Health?' *American Journal of Public Health*, 91, 6: 856–9.

Meyer, I. H., Rossano, L., Ellis, J. M. and Bradford, J. (2002) 'A Brief Telephone Interview to Identify Lesbian and Bisexual Women in Random Digit Dialing Sampling', *Journal of Sex Research*, 39, 2: 139–44.

Morris, J. and Rothblum, E. (1999) 'Who Fills Out a Lesbian Questionnaire? The Interrelationship of Sexual Orientation, Sexual Experience with Women and Participation in the Lesbian Community', *Psychology of Women Quarterly*, 23, 3: 537–57.

Morris, J., Waldo, C. R. and Rothblum, E. D. (2001) 'A Model of Predictors and Outcomes of Outness among Lesbian and Bisexual Women', *American Journal of Orthopsychiatry*, 71, 1: 61–71.

Morrison, C. and Mackay, A. (2000) *The Experience of Violence and Harassment of Gay Men in the City of Edinburgh*, Edinburgh: Scottish Executive Social Research.

Munro, S. (2003) 'Transgender Politics in the UK', *Critical Social Policy*, 23, 4: 433–52.

Naish, J., Brown, J. and Denton, B. (1994) 'Intercultural Consultations: Investigation of Factors that Deter Non-English Speaking Women from Attending their General Practitioners for Cervical Screening', *British Medical Journal*, 309: 1126–8.

Nardone, A., Frankis, J. S., Dodds, J. P., Flowers, P. N., Mercey, D. E. and Hart, G. J. (2001) 'A Comparison of High-Risk Sexual Behaviour and HIV Testing amongst a Bar-going Sample of Homosexual Men in London and Edinburgh', *European Journal of Public Health*, 11, 2: 185–9.

Nawyn, S. J., Richman, J. A., Rospenda, K. M. and Hughes, T. L. (2000) 'Sexual Identity and Alcohol-Related Outcomes: Contributions of Workplace Harassment', *Journal of Substance Abuse*, 11, 3: 289–304.

Nemoto, T., Operario, D., Keatley, J., Lei, H. and Toho, S. (2004) 'HIV Risk Behaviors among Male-to-Female Transgender Persons of Color in San Francisco', *American Journal of Public Health*, 94, 7: 1193–9.

Nemoto, T., Operario, D., Keatley, J., Nguyen, H. and Sugano, E. (2005) 'Promoting Health for Transgender Women: Transgender Resources and Neighborhood Space (Trans) Program in San Francisco', *American Journal of Public Health*, 95, 3: 382–4.

Newton, E. (1993) *Cherry Grove, Fire Island: Sixty Years in America's First Gay and Lesbian Town*, Boston: Beacon Press.

Noell, J. W. and Ochs, L. M. (2001) 'Relationship of Sexual Orientation to Substance Use, Suicidal Ideation, Suicide Attempts, and Other Factors in a Population of Homeless Adolescents', *Journal of Adolescent Health*, 29, 1: 31–6.

Nyman, D. (1991) 'A Deaf-Gay Man' (pp. 47–52), in G. Taylor (ed.), *Being Deaf: the Experience of Deafness*, Milton Keynes: Open University.

O'Connor, W. and Molloy, D. (2001) *'Hidden in Plain Sight': Homelessness amongst Lesbian and Gay Youth*, Edinburgh: National Centre for Social Research.

ONS (2001) *Counting Everyone In – The Big Challenge*, retrieved 15 November 2005 from http://www.statistics.gov.uk.

O'Toole, J. C. and Bregante, J. L. (1993) 'Disabled Lesbians: Multicultural Realities' (pp. 261–71), in M. Nagler (ed.), *Perspectives on Disability: Text and Readings on Disability*, Palo Alto, CA: Health Markets Research.

OPCS (1995) *1991 Census: General Report, Great Britain*, London: HMSO.

Parks, C. A. and Hughes, T. L. (2005) 'Alcohol Use and Alcohol-Related Problems in Self Identified Lesbians: Age and Racial/Ethnic Comparisons' (pp. 31–44), in E. Ettorre (ed.), *Making Lesbians Visible in the Substance Abuse Field*, Binghampton, NY: Haworth Press.

Parks, C. A., Hughes, T. L. and Matthews, A. K. (2004) 'Race/Ethnicity and Sexual Orientation: Intersecting Identities', *Cultural Diversity and Ethnic Minority Psychology*, 10, 3: 241–54.

Parsons, C. (2005) 'Exploring Transsexual Narratives of Identity Transformation: a Search for Identity', *The Psychology of Women Section Review*, 7, 2: 60–70.

Peel, E. (2001) 'Mundane Heterosexism: Understanding Incidents of the Everyday', *Women's Studies International Forum*, 24, 5: 541–54.

Penrod, J., Preston, D. B., Cain, R. E. and Starks, M. T. (2003) 'A Discussion of Chain Referral as a Method of Sampling Hard-to-Reach Populations', *Journal of Transcultural Nursing*, 14, 2: 100–7.

Peplau, L. A., Cochran, S. D. and Mays, V. M. (1997) 'A National Survey of the Intimate Relationships of African-American Lesbians and Gay Men: a Look at Commitment, Satisfaction, Sexual Behavior, and HIV Disease', in B. Greene (ed.), *Ethnic and Cultural Diversity among Lesbians and Gay Men*, Thousand Oaks, CA: Sage Publications.

Perry, J. (2004) *Is Justice Taking a Beating?* Retrieved 20 May 2005 from http://www.communitycare.co.uk.

Plumb, M. (1997) 'Butch Identity, Breast Reduction, and the Chicago Cubs: the Effect of Gender and Class on Lesbian Access to Health', in J. White and M. Martinez (eds), *The Lesbian Health Book: Caring for Ourselves*, Seattle: Seal Press.

Plumb, M. (2001) 'Undercounts and Overstatements: Will the IOM Report on Lesbian Health Improve Research?' *American Journal of Public Health*, 91, 6: 873–5.

Plummer, D. C. (2001) 'The Quest for Modern Manhood: Masculine Stereotypes, Peer Culture and the Social Significance of Homophobia', *Journal of Adolescence*, 24, 1: 15–23.

Ponse, B. (1978) *Identities in the Lesbian World: the Social Construction of the Self*, Westport, CT: Greenwood Press.

Potts, L. (2000) 'Why Ideologies of Breast Cancer? Why Feminist Perspectives?' (pp. 1–11), in L. K. Potts (ed.), *Ideologies of Breast Cancer: Feminist Perspectives*, Basingstoke: Macmillan.

Pringle, A. (2003) *Towards a Healthier Scotland: Working for Lesbian, Gay, Bisexual and Transgender Health*, Stonewall Scotland and NHS Scotland.

Pritchard, A., Morgan, N. and Sedgley, D. (2002) 'In Search of Lesbian Space? The Experience of Manchester's Gay Village', *Leisure Studies*, 21: 105–23.

Pugh, S. (2002) 'The Forgotten: a Community without a Generation – Older Lesbians and Gay Men' (pp. 161–81), in D. Richardson and S. Seidman (eds), *Handbook of Lesbian and Gay Studies*, London: Sage.

Rahman, M. (2004) 'The Shape of Equality: Discursive Deployments During the Section 28 Repeal in Scotland', *Sexualities*, 7, 2: 150–66.

Remafedi, G., French, S., Story, M., Resnick, M. D. and Blum, R. (1998) 'The Relationship between Suicide Risk and Sexual Orientation: Results of a Population-Based Study', *American Journal of Public Health*, 88, 1: 57–60.

Rich, A. (1983) 'Compulsory Heterosexuality and Lesbian Existence' (pp. 177–205), in A. Snitow, C. Stansell and S. Thompson (eds), *Powers of Desire*, New York: Monthly Review Press.

Richardson, D. (1994) 'Aids: Issues for Feminism in the UK' (pp. 35–51), in L. Doyal, J. Naidoo and T. Wilton (eds), *Aids: Setting a Feminist Agenda*, London, Taylor & Francis.

Richardson, D. (1996) 'Heterosexuality and Social Theory' (pp. 1–20), in D. Richardson (ed.), *Theorising Heterosexuality: Telling It Straight*, Buckingham: Open University Press.

Richardson, D. (2000) *Rethinking Sexuality*, London: Sage Publications.

Rivers, I. (2001) 'The Bullying of Sexual Minorities at School: Its Nature and Long-Term Correlates', *Educational & Child Psychology*, 18, 1: 32–46.

Rivers, I. (2004) 'Recollections of Bullying at School and Their Long-term Implications for Lesbians, Gay Men and Bisexuals', *The Journal of Crisis Intervention and Suicide Prevention*, 25, 4: 169–75.

Roberts, S. A., Dibble, S. L., Nussey, B. and Casey, K. (2003) 'Cardiovascular Disease Risk in Lesbian Women', *Women's Health Issues*, 13, 4: 167–74.

Robinson, A. and Williams, M. (2003) *Counted Out – the Findings from the 2002–2003 Survey Stonewall Cymru of Lesbian, Gay and Bisexual People in Wales*, Cardiff: Stonewall Cymru.

Robinson, C. M. (1997) 'Everyday [Hetero]sexism: Strategies of Resistance and Lesbian Couples' (pp. 33–50), in C. R. Ronai, B. A. Zsembik and J. R. Feagin (eds), *Everyday Sexism in the Third Millennium*, New York: Routledge.

Rosario, M., Schrimshaw, E. W. and Hunter, J. (2004) 'Ethnic/Racial Differences in the Coming-out Process of Lesbian, Gay, and Bisexual Youths: a Comparison of Sexual Identity Development over Time', *Cultural Diversity and Ethnic Minority Psychology*, 10, 3: 215–28.

Rosenblum, R. (ed.) (1996) *Unspoken Rules: Sexual Orientation and Women's Human Rights*, London: Cassell.

Rosenthal, M. S. (1997) *The Breast Sourcebook: Everything You Need to Know About Cancer Detection, Treatment and Prevention*, Los Angeles: Lowell House.

Rothblum, E. D. and Bond, L. A. (1996) 'Approaches to the Prevention of Heterosexism and Homophobia' (pp. ix–xix), in E. D. Rothblum and L. A. Bond (eds), *Preventing Heterosexism and Homophobia*, Thousand Oaks, CA: Sage.

Rothblum, E. D. and Factor, R. (2001) 'Lesbians and Their Sisters as a Control Group: Demographic and Mental Health Factors', *Psychological Science*, 12, 1: 63–9.

Rothblum, E. D., Factor, R. and Aaron, D. J. (2002) 'How Did You Hear About the Study? Or, How to Reach Lesbian and Bisexual Women of Diverse Ages, Ethnicity, and Educational Attainment for Research Projects', *Journal of the Gay & Lesbian Medical Association*, 6, 2: 53–9.

Rubin, G. S. (1993) 'Thinking Sex: Notes for a Radical Theory of the Politics of Sexuality' (pp. 3–44), in H. Abelove, M. A. Barale and D. M. Halperin (eds), *The Lesbian and Gay Studies Reader*, London: Routledge.

Russell, C. J. and Keel, P. K. (2002) 'Homosexuality as a Specific Risk Factor for Eating Disorders', *International Journal of Eating Disorders*, 31: 300–6.

Rust, P. C. (1997) ' "Coming Out" in the Age of Social Constructionism: Sexual Identity Formation Among Lesbian and Bisexual Women' (pp. 25–54), in E. D. Rothblum (ed.), *Classics in Lesbian Studies*, New York: Haworth Press.

Ryan, H., Wortley, P. M., Easton, A., Pederson, L. and Greenwood, G. (2001) 'Smoking among Lesbians, Gays, and Bisexuals: a Review of the Literature', *American Journal of Preventive Medicine*, 21, 2: 142–9.

Sale, A. (2002) 'Back in the Closet (Confronting the Needs of Ageing Gay and Lesbian People)', *Community Care*, 1424, 30 May: 30–1.

Sanchez, J., Meacher, P. and Beil, R. (2005) 'Cigarette Smoking and Lesbian and Bisexual Women in the Bronx', *Journal of Community Health*, 30, 1: 23–37.

Saunders, D., Oxley, J. and Harvey, D. (2000) 'Gay and Lesbian Doctors', *British Medical Journal*, 320, 7233: 2–3.

Saywell, C., Beattie, L. and Henderson, L. (2000) 'Sexualised Illness: the Newsworthy Body in Media Representations of Breast Cancer' (pp. 37–62), in L. K. Potts (ed.), *Ideologies of Breast Cancer: Feminist Perspectives*, Basingstoke: Macmillan.

Scherzer, T. (2000) 'Negotiating Health Care: the Experiences of Young Lesbian and Bisexual Women', *Culture Health & Sexuality*, 2, 1: 87–102.

Schiller, N. G., Crystal, S. and Lewellen, D. (1994) 'Risky Business: the Cultural Construction of Aids Risk Groups', *Social Science & Medicine*, 38, 10: 1337–46.

Schwartz, M., Savage, W., George, J. and Emohare, L. (1990) 'Women's Knowledge and Experience of Cervical Screening: a Failure of Health Education and Medical Organization', *Community Medicine*, 11, 4: 279–89.

Scott, S. D., Pringle, A. and Lumsdaine, C. (2004) *Sexual Exclusion: Homophobia and Health Inequalities: a Review of Health Inequalities and Social Exclusion Experienced by Lesbian, Gay and Bisexual People*, London: UK Gay Men's Health Network.

Seidman, S. (2002) *Beyond the Closet: the Transformation of Gay and Lesbian Life*, New York: Routledge.

Seidman, S., Meeks, C. and Traschen, F. (1999) 'Beyond the Closet? The Changing Social Meaning of Homosexuality in the United States', *Sexualities*, 2, 1: 9–34.

Sell, R. L. and Petrulio, C. (1996) 'Sampling Homosexuals, Bisexuals, Gays, and Lesbians for Public Health Research: a Review of the Literature from 1990 to 1992', *Journal of Homosexuality*, 30, 4: 31–47.

Selvin, B. (1993) 'One in Three Lesbians Risks Death from Breast Cancer', *The Guardian*, 6 February: 11.

Seneviratne, S. (1995) '. . . And Some of Us Are Older' (pp. 108–29), in V. Mason-John (ed.), *Talking Black: Lesbians of African and Asian Descent Speak Out*, London: Cassell.

Sexuality Matters (2005), *Leicester Lesbian, Gay and Bisexual Community Strategy*, Leicester.

Shakespeare, T. (1999) 'Coming Out and Coming Home', *International Journal of Sexuality & Gender Studies*, 4: 39–51.

Shakespeare, T., Gillespie-Sells, K. and Davies, D. (1996) *The Sexual Politics of Disability: Untold Desires*, London: Cassell.

Shilts, R. (1987) *And the Band Played On: Politics, People and the Aids Epidemic*, London: Penguin.

Simpson, M. (1994) 'Parading It: a Revisionist History of Homosex since Wolfenden' (pp. 262–74), in E. Healey and A. Mason (eds), *Stonewall 25: the Making of the Lesbian and Gay Community in Britain*, London: Virago.

Skinner, C. J., Stokes, J., Kirlew, Y., Kavanagh, J. and Forster, G. E. (1996) 'A Case-controlled Study of the Sexual Health Needs of Lesbians', *Genitourinary Medicine*, 72: 277–80.

Smith, T. W. (2002) 'The Hidden 25 Per Cent: an Analysis of Nonresponse on the 1980 General Social Survey' (pp. 108–25), in D. de Vaus (ed.), *Social Surveys: Sage Benchmarks in Social Research Methods*, London: Sage.

Solarz, A. (ed.) (1999) *Lesbian Health: Current Assessment and Directions for the Future*, Institute of Medicine, Washington, DC: National Academy Press.

Solomos, J. (2003) *Race and Racism in Britain*, Basingstoke: Palgrave Macmillan.

Speer, S. A. (2005) 'The Interactional Organization of the Gender Attribution Process', *Sociology*, 39, 1: 67–87.

Speer, S. A. and Potter, J. (2000) 'The Management of Heterosexist Talk: Conversational Resources and Prejudiced Claims', *Discourse and Society*, 11, 4: 543–72.

Stanley, L. (1995) *Sex Surveyed 1949–1994: From Mass-Observations Little Kinsey to the National Survey and the Hite Reports*, London: Taylor & Francis.

Stevens, P. E. (1994) 'Protective Strategies of Lesbian Clients in Health Care Environments', *Research in Nursing Health*, 17, 3: 217–29.

Stevens, P. E. (1995) 'Structural and Interpersonal Impact of Heterosexual Assumptions on Lesbian Health Care Clients', *Nursing Research*, 44, 1: 25–30.

Stevens, P. E. (1998) 'The Experiences of Lesbians of Color in Health Care Encounters: Narrative Insights for Improving Access and Quality', in C. M. Ponticelli (ed.), *Gateways to Improving Lesbian Health and Health Care: Opening Doors*, Binghamton, NY: Haworth Press.

Stewart, W. (1995) *Cassell's Queer Companion: a Dictionary of Lesbian and Gay Life and Culture*, London: Cassell.

Taylor, Y. (2005) 'Classed in a Classless Climate: Me and My Associates . . .' *Feminism & Psychology*, 15, 4: 491–500.

Terry, J. (1995) 'Anxious Slippages between "Us" and "Them": a Brief History of the Scientific Search for Homosexual Bodies' (pp. 129–69), in J. Terry and J. Urla (eds), *Deviant Bodies: Critical Perspectives in Science and Popular Culture*, Bloomington, Indianapolis: Indiana University Press.

Thompson, N. (1997) *Anti-discriminatory Practice*, Basingstoke: Macmillan.

Thompson, S. K. and Collins, L. M. (2002) 'Adaptive Sampling in Research on Risk-Related Behaviors', *Drug and Alcohol Dependence*, 68, 57–67.

Tiemann, K. A., Kennedy, S. A. and Haga, M. P. (1998) 'Rural Lesbians' Strategies for Coming Out to Health Care Professionals', *Journal of Lesbian Studies*, 2, 1: 61–76.

Townsend, P. and Davidson, N. (1979) *The Black Report: Inequalities in Health*, London: Penguin.

Troiden, R. R. (1989) 'The Formation of Homosexual Identities' (pp. 43–74), in G. Herdt (ed.), *Gay and Lesbian Youth*, New York: Haworth Press.

Valanis, B. G., Bowen, D. J., Bassford, T., Whitlock, E., Charney, P. and Carter, R. (2000) 'Sexual Orientation and Health: Comparisons in the WHI Sample', *Archives of Family Medicine*, 9, 9: 843–53.

Valentine, G. and McDonald, I. (2004) *Understanding Prejudice: Attitudes Towards Minorities*, London: Stonewall.

Vicinus, M. (1993) ' "They Wonder to Which Sex I Belong": the Historical Roots of the Modern Lesbian Identity' (pp. 432–52), in H. Abelove, M. A. Barale and D. M. Halperin (eds), *The Lesbian and Gay Studies Reader*, New York: Routledge.

Waites, M. (2000) 'Homosexuality and the New Right: the Legacy of the 1980s for New Delineations of Homophobia', *Sociological Research Online*, 5, 1: U39–U49.

Waites, M. (2003) 'Equality at Last? Homosexuality, Heterosexuality and the Age of Consent in the United Kingdom', *Sociology*, 37, 4: 637–55.

Wake, I., Wilmott, I., Fairweather, P. and Birkett, J. (1999) *Breaking the Chain of Hate: a National Survey Examining Levels of Homophobic Crime and Community Confidence Towards the Police Service*, Manchester: National Advisory Group/Policing Lesbian & Gay Communities.

Walker, L. (2001), 'Making Pretend Families: an Exploration of the Experiences of Lesbian Women in the North East Seeking Medical Help to Become Mothers', unpublished MSc Health Sciences: University of Northumbria.

Ward, J. and Winstanley, D. (2003) 'The Absent Presence', *Human Relations*, 56, 10: 1255–80.

Warner, M. (ed.) (1993) *Fear of a Queer Planet*, Minneapolis, MN: University of Minnesota Press.

Weeks, J. (1979) *Coming Out: Homosexual Politics in Britain, from the Nineteenth Century to the Present*, London: Quartet.

Weinberg, G. (1972) *Society and the Healthy Homosexual*, New York: St. Martin's Press.

Welch, S., Collings, S. C. D. and Howden-Chapman, P. (2000) 'Lesbians in New Zealand: Their Mental Health and Satisfaction with Mental Health Services', *Australian & New Zealand Journal of Psychiatry*, 34, 2: 256–63.

Welch, S., Howden-Chapman, P. and Collings, S. C. D. (1998) 'Survey of Drug and Alcohol Use by Lesbian Women in New Zealand', *Addictive Behaviors*, 23, 4: 543–8.

Wellings, K., Field, J., Johnson, A. M. and Wadsworth, J. (1994) *Sexual Behaviour in Britain: the National Survey of Sexual Attitudes and Lifestyles*, Harmondsworth: Penguin.

White, J. C. and Dull, V. T. (1998) 'Room for Improvement: Communication between Lesbians and Primary Care Providers', *Journal of Lesbian Studies*, 2, 1: 95–110.

Wilton, T. (1997) 'Healing the Invisible Body: Lesbian Health Studies' (pp. 212–27), in G. Griffin and S. Andermahr (eds), *Straight Studies Modified: Lesbian Interventions in the Academy*, London: Cassell.

Wilton, T. (1999) 'Towards an Understanding of the Cultural Roots of Homophobia in Order to Provide a Better Midwifery Service for Lesbian Clients', *Midwifery*, 15, 3: 154–64.

Wilton, T. (2000) *Sexualities in Health and Social Care: a Textbook*, Buckingham: Open University Press.

Wilton, T. and Kaufmann, T. (2001) 'Lesbian Mothers' Experiences of Maternity Care in the UK', *Midwifery*, 17: 203–11.

Winter, S. and Udomsak, N. (2002) 'Male, Female and Transgender: Stereotypes and Self in Thailand', *The International Journal of Transgenderism*, 6, 1. Available at http://www.symposion.com/ijt/ijtvo06no01_04.htm.

Wittig, M. (1988) 'The Straight Mind' (pp. 431–9), in S. L. Hoagland and J. Penelope (eds), *For Lesbians Only: a Separatist Anthology*, London: Onlywomen Press.

Yadlon, S. (1997) 'Skinny Women and Good Mothers: the Rhetoric of Risk, Control and Culpability in the Production of Knowledge about Breast Cancer', *Feminist Studies*, 23, 3: 645–77.

Yalom, M. (1997) *A History of the Breast*. London: HarperCollins.

Yip, A. (2005) 'Queering Religious Texts: an Exploration of British Non-Heterosexual Christians' and Muslims' Strategy of Constructing Sexuality Affirming Hermeneutics', *Sociology*, 39, 1: 47–65.

Young, R. M. and Meyer, I. H. (2005) 'The Trouble with "MSM" and "WSW": Erasure of the Sexual-Minority Person in Public Health Discourse', *American Journal of Public Health*, 95, 7: 1144–9.

Younge, G. (2005) 'How Stella Lost Her Groove', *The Guardian*, 22 July: 8–9.

Index